Healing the System

Praise for *Healing the System*

This book is the culmination of more than thirty years of learning about leadership and medicine. John is one of my life heroes and has had an amazing career. Not only is he an outstanding specialist in his medical field, but he has also played a role as a scientist, entrepreneurial businessman, and philanthropist while studying leadership science throughout every step of his journey. In *Healing the System*, you will glean his unique insights on improving healthcare for us all.

—Don Riling
Principle, Riling Resources LLC
Founder, Aquilla Leadership Institute, Rochester, NY

Dr. Hodgson is one of the greatest educators in medicine I've encountered in my training and even a better practitioner. It was hard for me not to notice what an amazing team he had on the first day. Everyone made me feel a part of the team. Of all the "little things" I've learned, there is one that sincerely hit home with me—how John went above and beyond to provide the best care possible for his patients. No matter their background, he treated each and every patient with utmost respect and passion. By reading *Healing the System*, you can experience the same innovative lessons!

—Nathan D. Schuerger, PA-C
Mercy Health, Lorain, OH

John Hodgson is incredibly bright, innovative, creative, and quality-focused. His personal integrity and commitment fit superbly with the healthcare organization. His willingness to contemplate novel solutions regarding physical resources, care delivery models, and human resource utilization sets a high standard for other leaders to emulate. His forward-thinking approach to most problems helped the group become more clinically productive and more service-oriented toward patients and referring physicians. Dr. Hodgson also has a personal work ethic that serves as an excellent role model for physician colleagues.

—Howard Grant, JD, MD
Principal, HRG Advisory Services, LLC
Former executive vice president and CMO, Geisinger Health System,
Danville, PA

I can state without reservation that John represents the best that the profession has to offer. As an administrator, each year the SCAI president is my partner in leading the organization in terms of personnel, financial management, and administration. Having served with nine SCAI presidents, I can state that John was equal to the best in leading the society in those respects. Lastly—but most importantly—John is a deeply compassionate caregiver, totally committed to excellence in patient care above all else.

—**Norm J. Linsky**
Executive director at the Pediatric and Congenital Interventional
Cardiovascular Society
Former executive director, Society for Cardiac Angiography and
Interventions (SCAI), Washington, DC

John Hodgson has the ability to generate leadership with the capabilities to attack the chaos in healthcare. He understands that superior coordination, information sharing, and teamwork across the many institution silos and disciplines are required if value and our patient outcomes are to improve. Because of his integrity, he understands shared responsibility that leads to collaboration vs. individual distinction.

—**Thomas Isaacson, MD**
Principle, TCI Cardiology Consulting LLC
Former chief of cardiology, Geisinger Wyoming Valley Medical Center,
Wilkes-Barre, PA

John Hodgson is a skilled interventional cardiologist, medical educator, innovator, and leader in healthcare. His knowledge, dedication, and professionalism are exceptional. His greatest strength may be in his ability to identify a need, envision a solution, and then make it happen! I have seen firsthand his ability to remain focused and flexible in the midst of dynamic clinical and business situations and deliver a positive result.

—**Laurie Harris, MSN, NP**
Manager, American Express Phoenix Wellness Centers, Phoenix, AZ

John is a very special individual—a constant innovator who is deeply committed to the medical profession and improving patient care. He is always using his God-given talents for the betterment of humanity. This has been his lifelong calling, with this book clearly being the intersection of these passions.

—**Seth Fischer, MD, FACC, FACP**
Chief of staff, medical director, Heart Failure and Cardiac Rehabilitation
Geisinger Wyoming Valley Medical Center, Wilkes-Barre, PA

John brings an amazingly broad knowledge base that includes years of medical, administrative, teaching, and business experience. He addresses key issues facing healthcare providers today. John's wisdom regarding teamwork, the integrity of character, and restoring broken processes through better communication is desperately needed. He points the way to a restoration of compassionate care as a primary goal of healthcare. He also advocates for a culture that fosters a restoration of community and healthier lifestyles for healthcare providers.

—**Joseph Daltorio**
Senior Pastor, River of Life Church
Board of trustees, Messenger International, Hudson, OH

In *Healing the System*, Dr. Hodgson correctly describes the flaws and inefficiencies within our medical system. The system is slowly crumbling at the foundation as physicians and nurses succumb to burnout and many leave the profession entirely. The prologue is a true day in the life of an attending physician, and it should worry you. While I trained with John for seven years, he continually fostered the principles described in this book with a common goal to provide efficient and excellent healthcare to patients. I have personally seen him have an impact on trainees, nurses, hospital leadership, and other hospital staff. I suggest not just hospital administrators but everyone read this book to learn the tools needed to rebuild our broken medical system. The pandemic should have illustrated just how healthcare affects us all, not just those within it.

—**Marissa Edmiston, MD**
Associate professor of medicine, Case Western Reserve University School of Medicine
Medical director, Cardiac Stepdown, MetroHealth Medical Center, Cleveland, OH

Healing the System is a book well worth the time to read and carefully consider the reality of the problems we face in healthcare. It contains some extremely practical and, indeed, pragmatic approaches to resolving or lessening the dysfunction. John has lived "where the rubber meets the road" for his entire professional career—he has been there and done that. I have had the honor of earning his friendship since 1987, when we first met. His integrity, leadership, humbleness, dedication, and competence have made him an extraordinary physician and human being. I strongly urge everyone from patients to practicing providers to healthcare administrators to national leaders to dig into this outstanding, detailed, and practical work.

—Lorick Fox, MPAS, PA-C, AACC
Distinguished fellow, American Academy of Physician Assistants
Associate, American College of Cardiology, Chester, VA

I've studied how to foster positive change for a large portion of my life, and I can say with confidence that Hodgson's book is a gift to the healthcare community. He identifies needed shifts in practice to create long-lasting improvements in the world of modern medicine. His action steps, if implemented, would foster a healthier, empowering environment for both providers and patients. Dive in and be refreshed.

—Rob Hoskins
President of OneHope, Pompano Beach, FL
Co-author of *Change Your World: How Anyone, Anywhere Can Make a Difference*

Healing the System

A prescription for rejuvenating
the heart in healthcare

John McB. Hodgson, MD

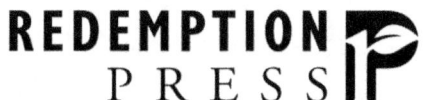

Published by Redemption Press, PO Box 427, Enumclaw, WA 98022.
Toll-Free (844) 2REDEEM (273-3336)

Redemption Press is honored to present this title in partnership with the author. The views expressed or implied in this work are those of the author. Redemption Press provides our imprint seal representing design excellence, creative content, and high-quality production.

The author has tried to recreate events, locales, and conversations from memories of them. In order to maintain their anonymity, in some instances the names of individuals, some identifying characteristics, and some details may have been changed, such as physical properties, occupations, and places of residence.

ISBN 13: 978-1-64645-560-7 (Paperback)
978-1-64645-559-1 (ePub)
978-1-64645-558-4 (Mobi)

Library of Congress Catalog Card Number: 2022909780

To my loving and unwaveringly dedicated wife, Dinah, who has been my constant support and best cheerleader. It has been a fantastic journey with you by my side, one I could never have done alone! And to my three wonderful children who love and honor me despite the many hours I spent away from them, the missed parties, and the absent dinners. Matt, Chris, and Catie, I am so proud of you and excited to walk with you as your own journeys are written!

Contents

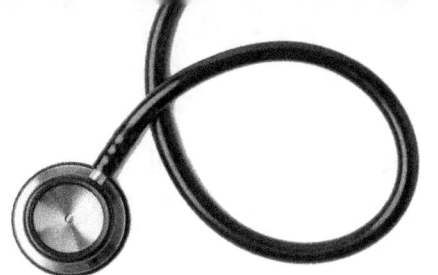

Foreword

We were just coming for a short visit.

My wife, Cheryl, and I arrived in Cleveland, Ohio, to spend a few days with some friends of ours who had recently started a new church. They had arranged for us to stay in the home of a family that was one of their members: a cardiologist, his wife, and their three children.

Dr. John Hodgson and his wife, Dinah, warmly welcomed us into their home. During those few days, we enjoyed some wonderful hospitality and great conversations about things that were mutually important to us, our families, and the world around us. Little did any of us know that those few days would launch a friendship that is finishing up its third decade!

Over the years, our kids interacted at youth camps, while John and Dinah joined us in several opportunities that our leadership group offered. They participated eagerly in events designed to build character, relationships, and leadership skills.

As time passed, I learned more about my friend John. Between the depth of his education and the breadth of his experiences, he was certainly one of the smartest and most accomplished men I had ever met. Since graduating from medical school in 1978, he has served tens of thousands of patients in ten states around our country, worked for a year in Germany, been a volunteer physician in countries around the globe, and been a guest lecturer/proctor in many more settings.

John and I often find ourselves in deep and meaningful conversations. It may be about places in our lives where we need to grow and develop. At times, it is about how to be better husbands and fathers. Other times, it is about our vocations and a desire to make a real impact—a generational difference—where we find ourselves working in society.

The latter brings me to this book.

I've heard it said by leaders around me that if you put good people in a bad system, the system wins every time. In my own experience, working with leaders in various vocations, I've found this to be 100 percent true! A bad system minimizes people's value and their unique contributions, reducing them to feel like they are just part of a machine. A bad system hinders healthy relationships and effective teaming toward one purpose. The system's red tape becomes increasingly frustrating and demotivating, and it remains hopelessly stuck in a scheme and structure that produces the same results year after year.

So how is it possible to change a system, making it more productive when it comes to its products and services and more life-giving for the people working within it?

Wisdom.

One of the things both John and I have learned over the years is that we need wisdom when it comes to leading our families, the life challenges that we are facing, and figuring out solutions within our vocations. We have both discovered that our good educations and broad experiences can only take us so far. To go further, we need wisdom. The basis for John's wisdom is founded on Judeo-Christian principles and practices that can bring about genuine transformation. Over our years of working together, I have watched John gain wisdom. In my own experience of four and a half decades working to create transformation on local, national, and international fronts, I have found that people are the key to change!

John understands this core piece of wisdom. In the pages of this book, John uses words like *community, connectedness, teaming, honor, humility, integrity,* and *accountability*—all of which have to do with the quality of one's character and a focus on one's relationships. People with good character who tend their relationships well can be fully counted on and trusted! People serving on teams using their unique strengths and pulling together as one can transform systems so that everyone can benefit.

As you read *Healing the System*, I'd encourage you to be open to laying aside what has already been tried and consider instead what still can be done. Think where you have found yourself snagged by the system and how the solutions John is proposing could be implemented where you work. Most importantly, be honest and reflect on where change may need to come within you or within your relationships. In doing so, you can be part of the solution, leading the charge toward change!

Dave Buehring
Founder and president, Lionshare Leadership Group,
Brentwood, TN

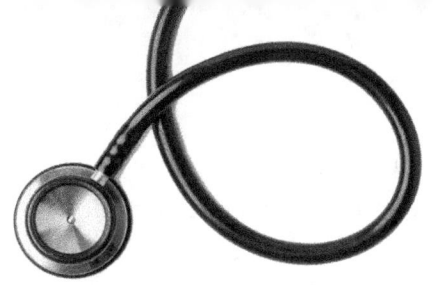

What's the Problem?

D r. Hall exits the elevator to the third-floor intensive care unit (ICU), carefully balancing his coffee mug while trying to badge swipe the door and keep his computer bag from spilling its contents to the floor. Carole, the charge nurse for the day, nods hello as he perches his mug on the nurse's station while sliding his computer bag under the desk. "Morning, Carole," he says, motioning to the room across the corridor. "How is Mrs. Chaudhry today?"

Carole's eyes widen. "Oh, she must be new."

One of the residents is sitting next to Carole, and Dr. Hall catches his eye while struggling to read his name badge. "Dr. Jackowitz," he asks tentatively, "what can you tell me about patient Chaudhry?"

"Oh, I'm new today; I'll have to check the computer."

Turning around, Dr. Hall sees Tom saunter up the hall. Tom (Dr. Green) is the cardiology fellow assigned to the ICU this week. Hoping for some relief, Dr. Hall asks him about Mrs. Chaudhry. A blank stare tells him Dr. Green will be of little help this morning. Addressing Paula, the unit housekeeper, Dr. Hall rolls his eyes and mutters, "I guess I will be on my own again today," knowing full well that Mrs. Chaudhry has been a patient on the unit for more than two days. Paula, who has worked there for fifteen years, nods slightly and smiles. She appreciates that Dr. Hall always says hello when he passes her.

I could be Dr. Hall, a tenured, full professor of medicine and the attending physician in the intensive care unit at a large teaching hospital. I have lived this scenario almost daily. I arrive at 7:50 a.m. armed with a list of patients given to me by the computerized electronic health record (EHR) and look for my team, which includes multiple residents (doctors doing further hospital training, typically for three years), fellows (doctors doing subspecialty training for two to three years), medical or other professional students, nurses, aides, and unit clerks. Frustratingly, it is very likely I will be the only person consistently providing care for an extended period, perhaps seven to fourteen days. All the other team members will be present only intermittently. When rounds start at 8:00 in the morning, I do not know which residents or how many will be present. Their schedules and the work-hour rules mandate that they have to go home at a certain time, have a day off, or switch rotations midweek. The residents who are there may have never met their patients before.

In some cases, three different resident team members will be responsible for one patient during a twenty-four-hour period. If this sounds like shift work, you are correct. To make matters worse, the assignments are shuffled each morning to ensure equal numbers of patients are assigned to each resident. Thus, the resident who cared for Mrs. Chaudhry yesterday may be assigned to a different patient today.

Nursing assignments are likewise variable. While there may be a charge nurse, they typically rotate between doing this job and caring for patients at the same time. They are not expected to know all the patients either, as their charge responsibilities relate mainly to staffing and scheduling. Some staff nurses work eight-hour shifts, some twelve-hour shifts, some nights only, some five-day weeks, some four-day weeks, and so on. Again, under the guise of being fair, nursing assignments are shuffled so that the same nurse does not have to care for the same very-ill patient for multiple days.

Unlike in years past, the unit clerks don't actually work for your unit anymore. They are part of a pool that helps multiple units, and they may not even be located near your unit! If a patient's family member calls when the computer is down, they will be unable even to tell the family member if the patient is still in the hospital.

Every day, I gird myself for what has become all too expected. When I ask how the patient is doing, four people head to the computer to see if there is any information. No one has actually talked to the patient yet. The resident may know the lab values drawn today but cannot tell me if they are different from yesterday. And so it goes, for fifteen patients.

While there is a large "team" caring for the patients on paper, it is hardly a situation where I thrive as a provider. Frustration and fatigue accelerate throughout the week-long assignment, and my excitement about my chosen career languishes in the reality of the dysfunctional system. As the attending physician, I am legally responsible for the patient and directing their care. Other than me, there is little consistency in the care delivered to the patient. Most members of the "team" are just trying to get through their assigned shift as smoothly as possible. Except for me, the other players are expected only to work their shift; another player will be assigned to relieve them after that.

I have seen this same scenario play out in the smaller community hospitals I have worked in as well. Today, I may be assigned to cover hospital consult patients. When I arrive (again, with my computer list), I try in vain to find anyone who might actually have information about the patient. Often, they were admitted overnight by a "nocturnist" or, in some cases, by a telemedicine provider. The hospitalist on-site today has not seen them. As in the teaching hospital, the nurses are on varied shifts, so they may not have handled that patient yet. Typically, the EHR notes are seven pages long (if you are lucky), with only one or two lines actually describing the medical decision-making at the time of admission. Since they are not required to be done for twenty-four hours, the history and physical (H&P) may not be written yet, so again, it falls to me to figure out what is wrong and how to treat the patient. I truly desire to get a handle on the issues, but I feel the tug of the other scheduled patients waiting for me in the clinic, not to mention the other procedures I have to perform. And if that isn't enough, the three new consults I'm there to see are expecting my attention!

Do these scenarios feel familiar to you? As a healthcare provider, have you experienced frustration and fatigue with an impersonal, administrative-heavy system where you don't feel your opinion matters? Do you feel powerless to effect change? I certainly have! But I now believe these issues can be addressed without significant expense or a major system overhaul!

It has taken me some time to write this book. In large part, this is because I have been mired in the problems, which I will outline, affecting medical care delivery today. I have started and stopped on a number of occasions, often feeling too tired or too frustrated to get my thoughts down on paper. Despite my frustrations, I've spent my adult professional life searching for answers to problems that have vexed my colleagues and me.

This is not a book about physician burnout but about reempowering healthcare providers to do the things they love to do—care for patients, solve problems, influence the delivery system, and have an enjoyable, empowering environment to work in. The message in this book will encourage physicians and other healthcare delivery professionals to create an environment and culture in which *everyone* can thrive by providing practical steps for positive change. As a colleague, it is also my intention to challenge healthcare administrators and system managers to appreciate the concepts outlined here and integrate them into how they design and manage delivery systems.

Part one will deal with *how we got here*. We will briefly review some of the major changes affecting the healthcare delivery system over the past forty years and why they have not always improved the delivery of care to our patients. In part two, I'll introduce *five fundamental areas that deserve special focus if we want to heal the system*. I have called them T.E.A.C.H.: Teaming, Equity, Administration, Community, and Honor. We will explore how simple changes in each of these fundamental areas can result in the reempowerment of healthcare providers. In Part Three, I will tell you about some key areas providers must personally work on if they want to become *effective leaders in the healthcare system*. The final part, part four, is my take on *what it would look like if some of these changes were implemented*—a futuristic, fictional scenario that I believe is easily attainable using suggestions from this book.

I trust that my words will resonate with you, the healthcare provider, to rejuvenate your heart and give you hope for a future where you can truly thrive as you practice medicine.

Part One
How Did We Get Here?

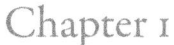

Chapter 1

What Changed?

U nless you were trained more than thirty years ago, you might be asking, *What's the issue?* From your perspective, practicing medicine has always been this way. You're probably wondering why some in this profession complain about the current system and think, *They just need to adapt!* But that's because you have never worked in the old system, where healthcare delivery was more of a mission and less of a business, and you've likely never practiced medicine without Relative Value Units (RVU) or Current Procedural Terminology (CPT) codes. Although the Accreditation Council for Graduate Medical Education (ACGME) requires training regarding billing and coding during residency, very little attention is paid to these seemingly mundane issues in reality. So a bit of history is needed to communicate what has changed and how we got to where we are today.

The American Medical Association (AMA) first developed Current Procedural Terminology codes in 1966.[1] The first edition was developed to simplify and bring consistency to the description of procedures and services. They were intended to help providers describe what they did more easily so record clerks could understand. The codes had nothing to do with reimbursement. In 1970, the second edition of the codes expanded to five digits and began including lab tests. Not until 1983 were the codes tied to billing. In that year, the Health Claim Financial Administration (HCFA), now called the Centers for Medicare and Medicaid Services (CMS), merged CPT with its own

Common Procedure Coding System (HCPCS) and mandated that CPT codes be used for all Medicare billing. An American Medical Association editorial panel of sixteen (largely) physicians oversees the codification. Thus, what started as a mechanism to help providers speak a common language has become a requirement for billing and a prime mechanism for tracing provider activity both locally and at a national level.

Relative Value Units are a measure of value used in the CMS reimbursement formula for physician services. RVUs are a part of the Resource-Based Relative Value Scale (RBRVS), designed to value physician services and serve as a guide for reimbursement.[2] Until RVUs were developed, CMS paid for services at a "usual and customary" rate, which could be quite variable. In the mid-1980s, a large study was authorized by Congress and conducted by researchers at Harvard University and the AMA.[3] The purpose of this study was to estimate the relative amounts of work expended by a provider in rendering a specific service. The estimated work considers provider time, training, technical skill, mental effort, and psychological stress. In 1989, President Bush signed a bill implementing the RBRVS fee schedule. These new fees became effective in 1992. The AMA Specialty Society Relative Value Scale Update Committee, also known as the RUC, sets and revises the RVUs and makes its recommendations to CMS. The AMA receives millions of dollars annually for licensing and to maintain the RVU/CPT system.

While the majority of providers agree to receive compensation for their activities based on the RVU/CPT system, you should understand that any provider can opt out of the system. At that point, the provider is free to charge whatever fee they would like, but they cannot charge patients insured by CMS. A number of super-specialized (especially aesthetic) providers, or concierge providers, have gone this route. Since CMS is such a large payer for most practitioners, opting out of caring for this patient population does not make sense. Importantly, once you opt out, you can never opt back in.

While a codified system certainly sounds like a good idea, there have been unintended consequences. CMS calculates the fee schedule from the RVU and CPT codes using a dollar amount conversion factor. Unfortunately, the conversion factor has not increased with inflation.[4]

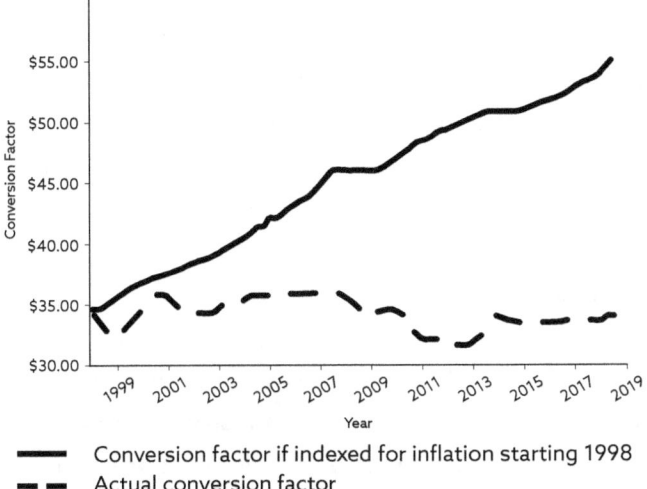

Figure 1. CMS conversion factor failure to keep pace with inflation. (Adapted from American College of Surgeons)

As figure 1 demonstrates, the conversion factor has actually declined rather than kept up with inflation. Thus, providers are paid less every year for the same effort in current dollars. Given this fact, it is easy to understand that providers would need to increase the number of billing episodes to maintain provider compensation with declining reimbursement. Whereas we used to be able to spend almost as much time as we needed with a patient to understand and diagnose their issues fully, we are now constrained to ten- to twenty-minute appointments and no more. Further discussion of a new patient concern requires a separate visit and a separate billing episode. We now see more patients in less time while having greater documentation requirements and an increased scope of medical issues to deal with. Needless to say, for those of us who began practicing before the mid-1990s, the impact of this on the way we interact with our patients has been profound. Those of you trained more recently are not fully aware of what our profession gave up as CMS ratcheted down reimbursement, so let me give you a picture of what it used to be like pre-1990s.

My first job after residency was at a large VA medical center in 1985. I have no recollection of doing any billing activity. If that did occur, it was abstracted from our progress notes and procedure reports by someone I never heard from. Little did I know then that it was a luxury to be able to focus on delivering patient care for as long as I needed and document my thoughts in the chart (with a pen!). I also had ample time to teach residents and fellows, spend two to three days per week doing research in an animal facility and with my patients, and publish and lecture around the world. I often performed procedures with a colleague by my side, knew my lab staff and research technicians, and even the fellows and their families. If I was working too hard (and I was), it was my own doing as I was striving to build my academic career. It was not because my medical director or hospital administrator pushed me to increase my clinical volume of procedures or visits.

When I moved to a large university academic center in 1989, I was still able to build and operate an animal facility, perform clinical research, train fellows and PhD students, participate in new hospital construction planning, and travel the world presenting my research findings. But as you might expect from the timing of the new CMS fee schedule, things were changing. The hospital became less and less willing to share resources if it involved research rather than clinical billing events. My "protected" time became scarce. If I wanted protected time, I had to find outside funding for my salary. Whereas presenting research on behalf of the university had been seen as a nice bonus for the university's reputation, my travel days became increasingly limited and questioned. By the end of the 1990s, if I wanted to travel for a presentation, I felt compelled to make up all clinical time by working extra on-call shifts. The protected time for research activities eventually vanished. My ability to support research nurses and technicians also vanished. Unfortunately, my days became increasingly filled with clinical activity and billing experts who frequented the department and schooled us on the necessity of proper billing documentation. We had moved from a mission-driven culture to a business-driven culture.

It is interesting to note that many hospitals were founded as religious outreaches to the communities. Catholic orders of nuns established huge numbers of healthcare facilities. In fact, the Roman Catholic Church is the largest non-government provider of healthcare services in the world.[5] This is especially true in developing nations. Many other hospitals were founded as local institutions (city or county) dedicated to serving the poor and needy. Whether religious or non-faith-based, most hospitals founded in the 1800s and 1900s were devoted to providing compassionate care, not generating income.

> Rather than being practitioners of the mission to serve the poor and ill, we have become the mechanism to ensure sufficient income and financial viability.

Over time, there has been a steady movement toward generating operating income from service fees. Charity and public funding have been insufficient to support the modern facility. To gain economies of scale, there has been massive consolidation such that locally responsive facilities are now a minority. Regulatory requirements have exploded. Legal risk has exploded. Medical complexity has exploded. Competition has overshadowed cooperation. To be sure, many hospitals still have written statements of values that reflect their founding missional principles, but the culture has shifted to a business and regulatory focus. Rather than being practitioners of the mission to serve the poor and ill, we have become the mechanism to ensure sufficient income and financial viability.

Enough about the old days for now. I feel it is important for us to realize that times have changed. I will share more experiences and contrasts from the past, but I want you to know that what we experience in current practice has not always been this way. And to be certain, I believe it does not have to *stay* this way. My goal for this book is to share how I think each of us working in healthcare can make small changes that will reshape our culture back to the mission without a major overhaul in the system or financial ruin.

Wouldn't it be great to be excited about coming to work each day and feel fulfilled that you have truly helped your patients after each visit? It used to be that way, and it can be again.

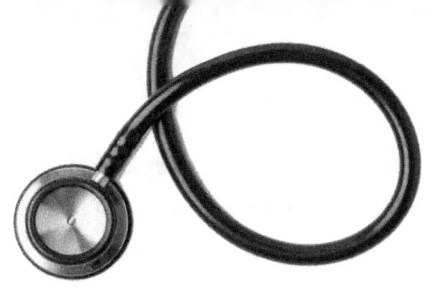

Chapter 2

Why Healthcare Providers Feel Stressed, Frustrated, and Depressed

The topic of healthcare delivery system structure is beyond the scope of this book, but I need to outline my working definitions to be applied throughout this discussion. It is important to state outright that healthcare providers are key to the healthcare delivery system. It is impossible to legally administer care to the patients without them, for all patient care requires a provider order. I do not mean that healthcare providers should be exalted or given unfettered authority; however, there is a need to recognize that they have a central role to play in the delivery system.

In modern healthcare systems, the consumers are the patients, their families, and in some cases, the referring physicians. While at times limited by insurance requirements, patients are generally free to determine where and from whom they obtain their healthcare. Therefore, an effective delivery system needs to be accessible and responsive to patients' needs.

The primary personnel required for a healthcare delivery system are the healthcare providers, including physicians, nurse practitioners, and physician assistants, who are extensively trained, licensed, and credentialed. Whether in an outpatient office or an inpatient hospital setting, all healthcare delivery requires the direction of a licensed provider. The hospital facility cannot function without engaged providers caring for patients, though they probably wish they could. And the hospital system doesn't direct the care for patients—providers do! All the other professionals in the system are part of the team facilitating the care directed by the providers. Nurses, aides, laboratory and radiology technicians, housekeeping, and maintenance workers all support the patient care prescribed by the provider.

The ultimate goal for a healthcare system is to deliver excellent care in a compassionate, effective manner to the consumers. This requires a team effort involving the healthcare providers in significant, meaningful roles.

Goal: To deliver excellent care compassionately and effectively. Requires a team effort.
Consumers: Patients, families, referring physicians. The system must be accessible and responsive to patient needs.
Healthcare Providers: Physicians, NPs, PAs. All care requires direction from the provider, licensed, board-certified, and credentialed, and the key to the Healthcare Delivery System.
Supporting Healthcare Personnel: Nurses, aides, laboratory and radiology technicians, housekeeping, and maintenance workers all support the patient care prescribed by the provider.

Table 1. Healthcare Delivery System Structure

Now more than ever, healthcare providers feel stressed, frustrated, and depressed with their jobs and the current system. According to a 2021 study by Medscape of over 12,000 physicians, 42 percent have reported feeling burned out.[6] While COVID-related stressors were cited as contributors, the factors listed as major determinants are well known to many of us, including bureaucratic overload, long work hours, lack of respect, and lack of autonomy (table 2).

Factor	% of respondents
Too many bureaucratic tasks	58
Spending too many hours at work	37
Lack of respect from administrators, employers, colleagues or staff	37
Insufficient compensation or reimbursement	32
Lack of control and autonomy	28
Increasing computerization of practice	28
Lack of respect from patients	27

**Table 2. What Contributes Most to Your Burnout?
(Adapted from Kane, "Death by 1,000 Cuts")**

From my own personal experience, four factors have been major contributors to provider discontent with the current healthcare delivery system.

- Providers feel increasingly minimized, dishonored, disrespected, and irrelevant.
- In the push for efficiency and throughput, the systems providers work in have become depersonalized and are isolating providers into one-person silos.
- Providers feel nitpicked about seemingly inconsequential administrative tasks and fill every moment of their workday with patient care (billing) activities.
- Providers feel a discontinuity between their intellectual curiosity and the pressure of maximizing care delivery.

Although my experience has been largely in an employed academic model, I have also worked in large community hospitals and small rural hospitals. I find the issues to be the same in all these settings. Many of my colleagues have shared their own stories with me, pointing to these same issues. The problem is pervasive and important. Let me share some reasons for the current dysfunction from my perspective.

Inadequate Acclimation and Systems Learning Time for Providers

Providers need time to acclimate to new surroundings and learn the systems of care before caring for patients. While I have had the opportunity to work in many different sizes of hospitals, I have dreaded the onboarding experience in all of them. It is usually disorganized and inadequate to prepare me to function effectively in providing patient care. Despite accepting a job several months in advance and having gone through a long credentialing process, I find the system does not appear to be ready for me when I arrive at the hospital!

Typically, on the first day, I am given a badge and receive training in the EHR, not from a provider but from an information technology (IT) expert who has never actually provided care for a patient using the system. Over the following two to ten days, I wait to get office keys, wait to have my badge reprogrammed to allow me into the areas that I predictably need access to, wait to get my name on the office door, wait to gain access to the parking lot, wait to get furniture in the office, wait to get a functional computer (that has the programs I need for my patient care loaded) in the office, wait to get business cards, wait to get a lab coat, wait to get a tour of the critical facility areas, and wait to get rudimentary training in the policies and procedures of the care delivery system. Despite the inadequate training and all of this waiting, I am expected to begin delivering patient care the same day I arrive at the hospital. In fact, at one new job, I arrived at 8:00 a.m. and was told I already had a patient waiting on the cardiac catheterization laboratory table for me! While most assume physicians are at the upper end of the intelligence-and-coping spectrum, we are still human and need time to acclimate to the new surroundings and learn the systems of care. No other business would hire an employee and expect them to interact with the client or consumer before being properly onboarded, would they?

Indeed, no hospital would ever consider onboarding new nurses or other staff without an organized orientation process lasting days to weeks. So why are providers any different? The lackadaisical onboarding process makes me feel minimized and dishonored and highlights the dysfunction in our system. Hospital administrators would be better served by a comprehensive approach, preparing long before the provider arrives. A few additional hours of provider-to-provider orientation would make the transition much more effective and allow the new provider to get up to speed quickly. Everyone would win, including the patients waiting for care!

Inadequate Training in the Electronic Health Record

Providers are now required to utilize EHR to document their findings and communicate with each other. Hospital administrators spend a lot of time encouraging physician engagement with the EHR, a constant battle for most systems. Complaints about the EHR are always near the top of any list of physician concerns. Our training in the systems has been inadequate, and using outside nonmedical consultants hired at huge costs has not proven effective.

Providers are typically instructed by nonmedical personnel who teach us the function of the buttons but have no fundamental understanding of how to utilize the system to investigate a patient's condition and construct a cohesive note demonstrating our medical decision-making and plans for the patient. Amazingly, I have rarely found significant peer coaching or peer instruction regarding optimizing EHR use. And I've never had any scheduled training from another provider regarding the ins and outs of using the EHR to care for patients efficiently.

That may not seem important, but there are numerous benefits to receiving practical training from other providers vs. nonmedical personnel. We could avoid many frustrating hours trying to "hunt and peck" to find things we need. We could also avoid delayed and incomplete note entries requiring reworking later. We could ensure that notes are complete, support the necessary billing requirements, and communicate essential medical information. We could raise the level of patient care and set a higher bar in communication from day one.

If training on one computer program isn't hard enough, many healthcare systems have one brand of EHR in the hospital and a different brand of EHR in the outpatient clinic. Compound that with another EHR system if you happen to practice at a different hospital, and you can appreciate why most providers are frustrated. I happen to like the EHR and have spent many hours exploring and tinkering. Most systems are quite customizable, and many customized features benefit the providers. But most new physicians get the same generic training and must start from square one to optimize the system for their particular mode of practice.

Providers are not afforded time to learn from other providers. Instead of interacting and talking with our colleagues, we now address a depersonalized computer, and support comes only from a remote, non-provider hospital IT system analyst. It does not have to be that way. At one large center where I served, I was able to work with our informatics department to preload all of the shortcuts and templates unique to our specialty. When a new colleague was onboarded, another EMR-savvy provider or I spent time with them. They learned how to efficiently use the system, our expectations for documentation, and any unusual quirks in the system. Simple provider engagement and sharing of customization during the initial training demonstrated respect for the new provider and ensured they could optimize patient care and billing in short order. It was a far more efficient process, despite the additional effort required.

Documentation Designed Only for Billing

Documentation should not fit billing needs only. Of course, billing is a necessary evil dictated by outside forces. A good chunk of time is spent redoing notes, adding more documentation, or changing the document to fit the billing needs. While it is important to document for continuity of care, getting paid/reimbursed by insurance, and so forth, the level of redos and rework leaves me feeling nitpicked and frustrated, knowing there is a discontinuity between my ability to explain my thought processes and the billing department's desire to maximize billing. I like to put short, unstructured notes in the chart that discuss important developments or major decision points. They can't be billed for, but in my opinion, they add more to patient care than the computer-generated tomes that compose most current documents. I feel professionally uncomfortable trying to enhance my documentation to fit a billing template.

This has also led to a syndrome of overdocumentation. Notes are often prepopulated with a completed review of systems and a routine physical exam. This is done to satisfy the system's desire for billing at the highest possible level. In my opinion, this is paramount to fraud. How often have you read a physical exam on a ninety-year-old patient that looks more like a sixteen-year-old high school athlete? How often do you think the admitting physician actually did tympanic membrane cold caloric testing? The result is often a note in excess of five pages with almost no information about thought processes. Unfortunately, while the physician is busy completing these billing-related elements, little time is spent documenting the thought that went into determining a care plan. Is it any wonder why most of these notes are never read by anyone but the billing office? Is it any wonder why continuity of care is difficult when it is hard to figure out what the last provider thought?

The chart (EHR) has the primary purpose of documenting provider findings and thoughts. Requirements that we detail system reviews for ten systems at two items per system, five physical exam components, and the like distract from the medical thought documentation. We need to get back to using the EHR to communicate, not just bill. It is well recognized that miscommunication during transitions of care is a problem. A 2012 Joint Commission report focusing on transitions of care estimated that 80 percent of medical errors involve miscommunication during handoff between medical providers.[7] Most EHR can be configured to enhance communication if a dedicated provider spends some time to create meaningful templates. A few hospital systems have excelled in this area, but many more need to get their providers involved in solving this issue.

Lack of Input for Purchasing Decisions

When a new hospital or clinic is designed, or new equipment is required, healthcare providers are typically included only tangentially.

That new space and the equipment in that space should be designed to facilitate delivery of care, and providers should have a say in recommending equipment and design features. In the past, providers were very involved. I recall in 1989 having weekly meetings to design, tweak, and optimize a new university hospital. I worked directly with the architects, engineers, and suppliers to ensure that the space and equipment would be optimal for delivering efficient, safe patient care. It was fun for me, but to be fair, not all providers want to be involved in these discussions. However, most like to be at least asked for their opinion.

It is important to remember that the hospital or the clinic is the factory where healthcare providers deliver care to the consumer. Others must also function in that space, but the other functions are designed to support the primary care delivery process. Too often, care providers are given cookie-cutter modules or leftover space in which to work. They are provided with shared offices and shared computers if they get an office at all. Purchasing decisions about the tools we need to do our jobs and the equipment we need to practice our profession are made by centralized purchasing administrators with little regard for our preferences.

I've had experiences in both being involved and not being involved in purchasing decisions, and the outcomes for each were far different. In one hospital where I was medical director of cardiology, a new telemetry system was purchased and installed with no apparent physician input. Once installed, it became clear that we could not access any of the patient analysis or summary screens from the patient care units—including the intensive care unit! To review the data required leaving the unit to visit the remote monitoring room personally. Efficient and safe patient care was actually reduced by obtaining the new equipment. Plus, it cost a lot more to reconfigure the system and fix a problem that could have been avoided by including providers in the initial acquisition process.

In a much larger system I worked in, the providers were able to redesign the new hospital plans to free up an entire floor while making patient care delivery more streamlined! This collaboration saved the hospital one million dollars since they no longer had to house another department off-site and could use the floor we no longer needed. By allowing direct physician interaction with equipment vendors, we were able to secure excellent pricing and upgrade several older systems as part of the negotiation. Physician negotiation with vendors is typically more productive than legal or administrative negotiation and more likely to end in purchasing systems that are optimal for patient care.

Lack of Time to Collaborate and Build Relationships

I remember with great fondness the daily 7:00 a.m. cardiology section meetings when I was a fellow at the University of Michigan. Everyone came—attendings, fellows, residents, medical students, and sometimes technicians and nurses. Every day was devoted to a different subspecialty area, such as ECG, catheterization, electrophysiology, imaging, or clinical diagnosis. One of us would present a case or two, and we would all discuss and learn together. I got to know my mentors and colleagues. I could look forward every day to a time of comradery and learning.

> We do not have to practice in an environment that feels increasingly hostile, isolated, and uncomfortable. Those days can be behind us..

When I interviewed for a job in the 1980s at the Sanger Clinic, the same process occurred there. The providers met each morning, talked about interesting cases, and established the team's workflow for the day. Needless to say, those days have long passed. Clinics now start earlier. Lab procedures start earlier. Rounds need to be earlier so that discharges can be accomplished earlier. Half the providers travel to outreach clinics and are not even in the building. Due to the American College of Cardiology COCATS (Core Cardiology Training Symposium) requirements in teaching institutions, we still have daily lectures. Still, it would be rare to have even the full complement of fellows and residents present, let alone any attending physicians besides the presenter! And in small community hospitals, you can forget any sort of case conference. The only time providers might discuss a case would be at a peer-review meeting investigating a serious complication.

I was fortunate to spend a year on sabbatical working in a catheterization laboratory at a heart hospital in southern Germany in the mid-90s. They were incredibly productive and efficient. But what I remember the most was sitting together for morning break, having coffee and pretzel bread, and then later spending forty-five to sixty minutes having lunch together. We would even go out after work and have a quick beer or spargel (asparagus.) Nowadays, we double book patients during the lunch hour, fit in some echo reading, or catch up on charts rather than having any downtime with our colleagues. The doctor's lounges, which used to be a nice place to relax and catch up, are now empty and barren. The sparse snacks that are sometimes stocked spoil before they are eaten. As we will discuss later, lack of relationships at work is a major detriment to workplace satisfaction. Healthcare providers understand the demands of the job when we enter the profession; however, to be continuously effective, healthy, and enjoying the work we do, we need to develop supportive relationships.

You may be able to identify with some (or all) of the examples I have given above. Hopefully, I have piqued your interest, so let's find solutions that can be easily applied and will yield huge benefits. We do not have to practice in an environment that feels increasingly hostile, isolated, and uncomfortable. Those days can be behind us.

Part Two

Healing the System

You would think in a book about healing our healthcare system, I would delve into many very complex solutions that would take countless administrative hours and millions of dollars to enact. But really, it's much simpler than you think. I've developed five fundamental concepts that will allow healthcare providers to thrive in their chosen profession. They are not expensive, nor are they difficult to implement. They are beneficial not only for providers but also for the health of the hospital system and, most importantly, for the patient's care. They just require a unified effort to institute. I have called them by the acronym T.E.A.C.H. I'll take you briefly through each concept, along with outlining some steps you can take, things to avoid, and some simple implementation tips for you or the department you work with.

- Teaming—Using a Team Approach (Ch. 3), Making Teams Work in Your Setting (Ch. 4)
- Equity—Encouraging Equity (Ch. 5)
- Administration—Involving Providers in Administrative Functions (Ch. 6)
- Community—Building Community for Connectedness (Ch. 7)
- Honor—Practicing Honor (Ch. 8)

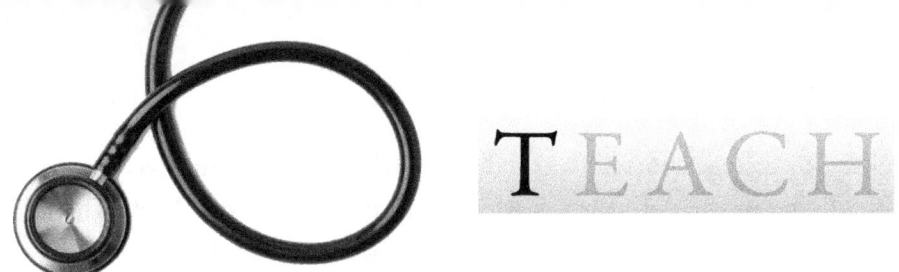

TEACH

Chapter 3

Using a Team Approach

Sally walked from the bus stop into a recently built neighborhood in the sprawling suburb of Oakwood, Ohio. The homes were pretty typical, the kind that seemingly pop up overnight once the developer gets approval. Like most of the other kids there, Sally and her brother were getting used to their first home, one their parents had dreamed of for years! It was a beautiful spring day, and the gaggle of kids streaming off the bus was excited to be outside. Jimmy, the de facto leader of the cool kids, was organizing a pickup baseball game. Sally ran home as fast as her legs could carry her to retrieve her mitt from the moving box labeled "sports stuff" still stacked in the garage. By the time she got back to the vacant lot, they were already picking teams for the first game of the neighborhood season. She waited nervously with some of the other girls, secretly hoping she would get the chance to show that she, in fact, did know how to play baseball. Despite being picked last, she was still happy to be on the team with Jimmy and her best friend, Sonja. But once she pitched the first inning, her place on the team was secured! Three up, three down! Her teammates cheered! All was right in the neighborhood.

From a very young age, all of us, like Sally, learn about teams. We learn that teams are groups of people who spend time together doing something fun or productive. We learn that it is natural and rewarding to be with others and work toward a common goal. It could be Little League baseball, neighborhood soccer games, school debate clubs, or college sports. I learned to ski when I was about five years old, living in the Adirondack Mountains of upstate New York. The school used to run a bus out to Snow Ridge so we could get in some skiing after classes ended. There were plenty of opportunities with an annual snowfall of over four hundred inches. Despite a broken leg at age seven, my passion for skiing continued through high school and into college. I was an accomplished skier, but nothing like my college friends, many of whom were also on the US Olympic team.

I just loved being on the college team with them. In those days, as long as you showed up for practice, you could be a member. (Of course, now it requires tryouts and invitation.) We were a close-knit group, often spending long evenings talking in the basement of the Outing Club while tuning our skis. I was not a particularly good racer, but it didn't matter; I was part of the team and was thrilled when my teammates did well. After college, something happened. For those of us who chose to pursue a healthcare career, goals became increasingly singular. It was no longer a team effort. There was no team helping you to get a good Medical College Admission Test (MCAT) score. Then with scores in hand, I competed with my classmates for the elusive acceptance to medical school. The same friends I used to enjoy studying and skiing with now threatened my future career. This process repeats at least twice for physicians, and for specialists three or four times as we strive for residencies and fellowships. All this competition, and we don't even have a real job yet!

As we enter our first real job, is it any wonder that the concept of teaming is long forgotten? We settle into our silos. As if separating the providers into silos isn't bad enough, the system separates us even further. In most institutions, nurses report to the nursing office, physicians to the medical staff office, and the administrators avoid us all! Nurses work on nursing goals, social and caseworkers on family and support issues, and physical and occupational therapists on their niches. Providers are often included with these other departments only to "encourage" them to keep the patient flow going or when things go wrong. The current system neither promotes nor supports cross-discipline teams.

The way we construct teams can lead to success or failure. A team will fail if it distributes responsibility so that no one is really in charge. Many medical teams do this by including multiple director-level members, none of whom is actually in charge. This type of team is often constructed to keep everyone involved or informed. Unfortunately, they are rarely empowered actually to advance the mission of the organization. Teams also fail due to a lack of continuity when the team is composed of "positions" rather than people. Positions can't develop effective teams; only people can. As the person filling the nursing supervisor role changes daily, so does the team dynamic. How can we establish personal trust and intimacy when players constantly change?

> The way we construct teams can lead to success or failure. A team will fail if it distributes responsibility so that no one is really in charge.

On the other hand, a successful team can lessen stress and workload by distributing tasks in an optimal manner. A successful team offers a collaborative effort by persons with different talents, all of whom have developed relationships with their teammates and are enabled to contribute. There is a reason why effective football teams do not have twelve wide receivers. Neither do effective football teams change players every set of downs. They work hard to form bonds between players of different positions to enable them to execute a common plan. Would not the same concept work in the delivery of healthcare? I think it would.

The Three Cs

Team success requires three things; I call them the three Cs: a captain, consistency (continuity), and a common goal. To be effective, teams must have all three Cs:

The Captain

Someone must be in charge. Whoever it is, it must be clear who they are, and they must exercise leadership over the rest of the team. While the captain does not necessarily establish the rules or the expectations, they certainly espouse them to the rest of the team. He or she oversees the activities of the team and is an active part of the team at the same time. I live in Cleveland, and I was fortunate to be there during the second "reign" of "King James." No one on the Cavaliers NBA basketball team questioned who the captain was: LeBron James! LeBron set the expectations (win a championship) and set the work ethic. He encouraged, counseled, and corrected his teammates. He kept them focused on the goal, and he expected them to be their best at all times. So, too, in the medical profession the physician must function as the captain. He or she must set the expectations and the tone. When this responsibility is taken away or is hampered, the team suffers, and the physician becomes less effective. While this is not a book specifically about leadership, it should go without saying that being the captain does not mean being dictatorial, divisive, or mean spirited. Any leader, whether in medicine or not, must use basic leadership skills to guide their team. Unfortunately, leadership skill training is *not* part of any medical curriculum. More about this later.

Consistency or Continuity

It is hard to have a team when the players shift every day. Teams must get used to one another; they must learn the team culture, the team expectations, and the team "flow." When new elements are added to the team, it takes time for everyone to adjust. When new elements are added daily, the team never coalesces. Let's look back at the Cavaliers basketball team in early 2016. The team was not working as well as expected. The championship goal was looking more elusive. Multiple trades were made in the late winter. For a while, the new team members did not play well. The Cavaliers continued to lose. But by late spring, they started to gel and work together. James encouraged this fledgling team all the way to the NBA Finals! To be successful, a team must be consistent. Further, a team is made of individuals, *not* titles or positions.

As the person filling any particular role changes daily, so does the team dynamic. It is a specific individual who lends their unique perspective to the team, understands the patient's history, and knows the strengths and weaknesses of the players on the team. Having a consistent individual filling the roles will improve efficiency, resulting in fewer patient care errors, better patient satisfaction, and a healthy, more enjoyable team dynamic. We will discuss the importance of culture for workplace satisfaction in a later section.

Common Goal

The common goal is an oft-overlooked component of teaming. Just as James defined the goal for the Cavaliers (winning the NBA championship), a team in the medical field must have a clear common purpose. While many hospitals have mission or vision statements, these are too far removed from the day-to-day teams. Every member of the team must be working for the same goal. That goal must be tangible, clear, consistent, measurable, and continually reinforced. Too often, the team members report to different managers and are evaluated by different metrics, creating conflicting agendas and performance needs. Plus, think about it from the team member's perspective, never knowing if they are hitting the goal. When we feel pulled in different directions, we will tend to take the path of least resistance rather than go out of our way to figure out the actual goals.

A common goal in daily patient care may seem obvious, but I suggest it is more complicated than it appears at first glance. While we would all like the patient's health to improve, other (often unspoken) forces threaten our goals every day. The emergency room may be busy and have patients waiting for admission, which puts pressure on the system to discharge patients rapidly. A self-employed man may have no insurance and is threatening to leave against medical advice for fear of a large bill. This confounds the delivery of care and calls for special financial and social expertise.

Also complicating matters is an unwritten expectation that everyone must participate for the entire time the team is meeting. This is not true; at times, the concept of divide and conquer is more appropriate. The team may have to split to care for an emergent patient need and continue routine patient rounds. This is still consistent with the overall goal of improving patient health. The nature of acute care is made up of unpredictable events, which can derail the most careful planning. The team needs to be aware of this and adaptable to accommodate these interruptions.

Outside of day-to-day care, system-wide goals can effectively encourage teams. I once worked for a large integrated healthcare organization. The entire organization had three to four major goals each year. Each department and division was required to outline several practical, achievable goals within each major goal topic. For the Cardiovascular Department, topics might include a quality initiative to reduce inpatient mortality after coronary surgery. Another topic might be to improve patient access to care. These goals were individually assigned (and agreed to) at the beginning of each year, and 25 percent of each employee's compensation was tied to accomplishing these specific goals. The majority of the goals required working in teams to execute. Administrators, nurses, physicians, and insurance providers were all working toward the same goals. Talk about alignment! I am not suggesting that monetary reward is the only way to align goals; however, having a vested interest is a strong motivator, and receiving compensation for meeting goals demands action.

Goals are not mission statements posted on a plaque in the entry lobby; rather, they are the tangible outcomes that affect patient care: lowering mortality after a heart attack or ensuring that every patient undergoing bypass surgery had forty key quality metrics accomplished. While the Joint Commission on Accreditation of Healthcare Organizations (JCAHO) has put forth some countrywide care goals, these are not enough. Specific, local system goals are needed to encourage team building, address specific deficiencies, and advance unique service offerings.

Steps You Can Take

Define the captain.
A single person needs to be in charge. Of course, this responsibility can be rotated if appropriate. For example, after a resident gets some experience, assigning them to be the captain can effectively help them develop their leadership skills.

Keep the team consistent as much as possible.
Teams need to be given priority when scheduling. If you are building a patient care team, ensure that the same physicians and nurses are assigned to the same patients each day until that patient is discharged. Continuity of care should be given priority, provided super-specialized services do not require a transfer of care. After caring for a patient in the intensive care unit during the critical part of their illness, continuing to care for them in a step-down setting is logical and satisfying. Far too often, once patients are no longer deemed critical, they are transferred to a different team that doesn't know them and one they do not trust. A recent trend in some new hospital construction is the ability of every bed to flex between ICU level care and routine floor care. This makes it easy for patients to stay with the same team. Patients love not being moved at 2:00 a.m., and it is rewarding to follow the patient's recovery and see them go home!

Provide continuity as the number one priority in meeting assignments.
If you are building a non-patient care team, it is just as important to have consistency. These could include the pharmacy and therapeutics committee, the quality review committee, or any other system or practice-level standing meeting. Meetings for these teams need to be prioritized, schedules need to be blocked, and, importantly, alternative patient coverage for providers needs to be arranged. If this is not done, provider attendance will always become secondary to the constant pull of patient needs. When I established a monthly counsel to advise the department, the provider members were always free of

other responsibilities surrounding the meeting times. The travel time necessary to attend was also blocked so that there were no obstacles to attendance. It makes no sense to include providers on a committee team if the meeting carries on just as easily without them.

Discuss and define the team goals.
This may include a basic foundational goal, such as effective, efficient, error-free patient rounds, with additional specific short-term goals, like reducing ventilator-associated pneumonia or reducing the length of stay by 10 percent in six months. For the larger system goals, sufficient time for discussion and revision needs to be allotted. Once everyone agrees to the goals, I encourage creating a memorandum of understanding. The old adage that the more familiar you are with a teammate, the more necessary it is to have it in writing applies here.

Provide orientation to new team members.
They need to be well versed in the expectations and culture. I am alarmed at how little attention is paid to this by healthcare providers. I suggest creating a one-to-two-page document that outlines the key goals and expectations. This can be given to all members and any new members who may join. An hour spent clarifying and discussing this document can get the team off on a good trajectory. Every resident working with me in the ICU gets a two-page handout that outlines my expectations.

Provide performance reviews that highlight the individual's contribution (or lack thereof) to the team goals.
Ignoring routine performance reviews creates many issues. First, it implies a lack of interest in the individual. If no review is ever done, the logical assumption is that one's contribution is of no concern or importance. Second, if a person is not meeting expectations, documented written reviews and corrective action plans are required if job termination is ever considered. Third, these sessions provide an excellent forum for education, encouragement, and career advice.

Have periodic reviews of the team performance and goals with an eye toward continuous improvement.
All teams have issues and bumps in the road. Having regular debrief sessions apart from the daily operation is important to work these out and encourage increased effectiveness.

Measure elements that the team is working on, make them public, and celebrate wins! In every setting, people attend to things that are being measured.
It is important to measure the team's effectiveness and set the expectation that there will be efforts to improve.

Review situations where bad outcomes occur.
Discuss how the team may have failed or could improve to prevent similar events in the future. Having the entire team participate can provide an atmosphere where everyone feels empowered to contribute to the discussion and suggest solutions.

Foster the concept of each member working at the "top of their license."
We should let people take on more responsibility and encourage them to do so. The captain needs to provide space for team members to take the initiative even if they fail at first. Assigning tasks only to those with proven expertise fails to foster development in the less experienced.

Expect excellence, participation, and accountability.
It is far easier to relax standards than to try to elevate them. Set expectations high and encourage the team to meet them. If a member falls short despite a good effort, then graciously allow them to reengage at a more comfortable level. After their orientation, my residents who arrive for rounds in scrubs are quietly sent home to dress appropriately. It never happens a second time.

Include the patient as part of the team!
Experiencing a patient's small successes or setbacks together makes the team more focused. Having the team present when good (or bad) news is presented will be meaningful to the patient and build the team's understanding of that patient's situation. Get patient and family feedback on how the team is serving them. This will be far more effective than reviewing mind-numbing Press Gainey patient satisfaction scores.

Things to Avoid

Don't have a team with multiple "captains" bringing varied views and expectations.
In the case of patient care teams, make every effort to have a system-wide expectation of how the team will function so that changes in provider captains will have minimal impact.

Try to avoid scheduling assignments to be fairer, rather than to provide patient/staff continuity.
While it may appear that caring for the same sick patient for multiple days is unfair, I have found it is easier than trying to learn about new patients from scratch. Our job is not to ensure equal numbers of patients on a list; our job is to ensure optimal patient continuity while minimizing opportunities for error. Unnecessary personnel switches must be avoided.

Avoid developing pools of employees in the name of efficiency.
I see this often with unit clerks, housekeeping, and scheduling. Someone assigned to no one in particular will likely be committed to no one in particular. Having consistent unit clerks and scheduling staff who know your unit or clinic and the standard procedures you have developed can make the team run smoothly. Similarly, a housekeeping employee assigned to your unit or area and whom you talk to and see every day will be much more likely to pitch in when things get busy and you have urgent needs.

Don't set up conflicting expectations from various managers or departments.

These system-related issues will need to be settled before you can have effective interdepartmental teams. Everyone needs to agree on priorities before the day-to-day interruptions begin. I have been the captain on teams where two nursing members were reassigned midmorning without notice. I have had resident physicians switch overnight with no notification. I have had daily resident schedules changed by the department head with no notification. Not only does it disrupt the team, but it is also disrespectful to the captain of the team.

Team members should be evaluated by their teammates, not just by unrelated managers from different departments.

The team should provide an important part of any employee evaluation they function as part of. Otherwise, the team is just something to be tolerated but not viewed as that important. Input from members belonging to different job functions can be very enlightening. This is similar to the "360" evaluations that have become popular.

Try not to have "token" charge nurses who are only in charge of staffing assignments.

Many are taking care of patients as well. In my experience, an effective charge nurse provides oversight to all patients and nurses on the unit. They know the whole situation and can anticipate problems in advance rather than just react to acute staffing needs. Of course, like all of us, they can pitch in to provide care for emergent or unusual situations, but that is not their primary role. An added benefit is that they have time to teach newer employees advanced skills and mentor them in their career development.

Failure to give responsibility and assign accountability to team members.

Setting clear expectations and holding members accountable is important for building an effective team. I have also encountered many situations where team members feel no responsibility to perform to my expectations. In most cases, this relates to the previously mentioned reporting structure. Regardless of which department hires the employee, they need to be a responsible member of the team and adhere to team expectations.

Don't allow bad outcomes to be overlooked or reported only to a computer database.

Most academic systems have some type of morbidity and mortality conference. In years past, we used to discuss many cases. Now, there is often only one case, and the meeting is used more for education than problem-solving. Only when a potential legal situation arises does a case get elevated for a root cause analysis. Discussing even mildly undesirable outcomes can provide opportunities for improvement and growth for the team.

Don't forget the patient.

They are not a room number or the "lady in the corner." They are the reason you have a job at all.

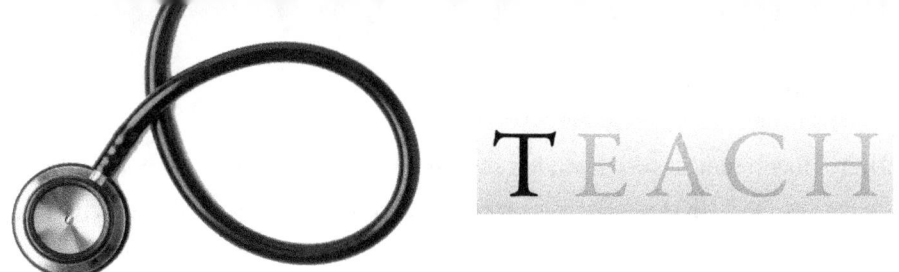

Chapter 4

Making Teams Work in Your Setting

I started the book with a description of what I call a bad team in a large teaching hospital. I propose that this type of team is bad because it is ineffective and in many cases leads to increased frustration and fatigue for providers. While there are many bodies to assist, there is only one person capable of effectively guiding the team, thus carrying all the weight. There are many healthcare delivery settings besides an academic hospital, so in this section, I will describe my experiences in other settings so we can explore how effective teaming could work in each one.

Community Hospitals

In contrast to a large teaching hospital, community hospitals in my experience are more likely to foster an effective team model. I have had the opportunity to work in varied hospitals with as few as twenty beds to as many as six hundred. Some have been located in rural towns and some in large cities; some were for-profit, some not-for-profit, and some publicly run. Let's imagine a scenario where I am the staff hospitalist physician at a community hospital. The team there is smaller, yes, but I have found that to be beneficial, in part because everyone understands their role, and their responsibility is clear. In addition to me, there are perhaps an advanced practitioner (physician assistant or nurse practitioner), the nurses, aides, the social worker and case managers, and the unit clerk. I may even have a scribe to assist with recording in the EHR.

There may be nurses with varied schedules; however, there is an active charge nurse who is not caring for patients, and the expectations on the charge nurse are different from those in many academic institutions. They are *expected* to know everything about the patients on their unit.

When I arrive, the charge nurse can easily give me a summary of how each patient is doing and who has the most pressing needs. The social worker and case managers round with me and provide valuable suggestions and solutions. At the bedside, both the advanced practitioner and the nurse will be with me and can answer any questions about the lab values, overnight patient course, and the like. They may also remind me of any orders or labs that are needed or overlooked. The unit clerk knows me and has already taken it upon themselves to send for outside records on new patients. Unit rounds proceed smoothly and efficiently. I have time to teach my colleagues as we discuss each patient. I also have time to talk to the patients and their families. My teammates hear these discussions and, therefore, are even better equipped to reinforce the treatment plan.

While there are fewer members, I suggest that this team is far more effective and will be more likely to provide the support needed to care for both the patients and the providers. All three Cs are present. The *captain* is the same, but now there is *consistency*; the same key persons will be there tomorrow and the day after that. Perhaps there will be two in each role, but the provider will know both, and they will both be oriented to the team. Comradery can be established. Patterns can be learned. Best practices can be implemented. Additionally, there is also a clear *common goal*, which is providing effective and efficient care. This goal is measured and promoted at all levels of the team. By the way, when I worked as a hospitalist in this environment, it was a wonderful experience!

Outpatient Clinics

Serial Processing Model

In a large hospital desiring efficient use of its outpatient exam space, there may be forty or more exam rooms in the outpatient wing servicing multiple types of physicians. The concept of a physician's personal office has been replaced by a factory or assembly line model. Think of it this way: There are many ways to exercise, but hiring a personal trainer to supervise you feels vastly different from just going to the gym and having the staff of the day tell you how to work the machines. A medical relationship is between provider and patient, not clinic and patient. These large clinics are staffed by multiple nurses and aides. They are assigned to the clinic, not to specific providers. They are trained to be multifunctional and interchangeable. At times, a provider may work with the same staff, but this is neither guaranteed nor even strived for.

The clinic has multiple providers. They use the generic clinic space based on an efficiently mapped-out strategy. On Mondays, it might be cardiology day; Tuesdays, pulmonary; Wednesdays, endocrine; and so on. You are assigned a certain number of rooms with little flexibility. If you want any special tools or literature in the clinic, someone will have to bring it specifically for your day. Patients typically check in at a separate desk with multiple clerks. They specialize in getting patients registered and checking on insurance and contact information, but they are not trained to know the providers or anything about what the providers do. Thus, there is a large, efficient team to help the clinic run smoothly. Unfortunately, this system is depersonalized for the patient, the staff, and the providers. The focus is on efficient patient throughput, not compassionate, effective patient care.

This type of clinic is set up for *serial processing*. Patients are moved through the system one at a time, attended by one person at a time. If the patient is late, has a problem with language or mobility, or needs extra time for a unique problem, the entire process stops. In fact, one clinic I worked in had the policy of canceling and rescheduling any patient who was ten minutes late! There is little capacity to handle the unusual or emergent in this system. Most likely, a sicker patient will be sent to the emergency department to be handled, as there is no ability to "stop the line" and attend to an issue in a clinic that uses serial processing.

When I worked in these clinics, I typically brought handouts detailing how I would like tasks to be completed. I had instructions for how to measure ankle brachial indices, how to take postural vital signs, and how to properly place the precordial leads for an electrocardiogram. I could not expect the staff to know these details unique to cardiology. I also brought patient handout information, or I preloaded a shelf with what I needed so I knew where to find it. If I was lucky, I might have two rooms assigned to me. During the time I was with patient A, patient B could be placed in the second room and initial screening performed. This at least limits downtime between patients. If I was unlucky, I had only one room, and we were back to serial processing again! I was never sure which nurse I should ask for assistance. I was unable to get in-office ancillary testing. All too often, I was told it must be scheduled at a different time or that there was no room to put the patient in for such testing.

If an advanced practitioner was there, they worked their own schedule, and I was competing with them for open rooms. I was typically behind schedule and left the clinic with incomplete charts. Some large clinics go a step further. The patient is not necessarily seen by the same physician at each visit. They are assigned to a medical team and seen by anyone from that team who is free. Physicians do not like this. Patients do not like this, and patient care suffers from a lack of continuity.

Not all of these large clinics are totally generic. At one heart, lung, and vascular service I worked in, we had a limited number of related providers but with considerably different clinic needs. Even within this relatively small group, we had general cardiology, electrophysiology, heart failure, vascular surgery, cardiothoracic surgery, general pulmonary, sleep medicine, and pulmonary hypertension divisions. As you might imagine, it was difficult for the staff to be expert in all of these disciplines, but it was certainly better than a totally generic model. Nonetheless, the serial processing issue was the same. In this type of clinic, I found the ability to effectively team was very difficult, as the clinic staff was never really part of any focused team.

This model lacks all of the key C components. There is no *captain*—the clinic is run by an administrative directive. There is no *consistency*, as the providers, room assignments, and practice types change daily. And it is hard to have a *common goal* when it changes daily. One way around this is to bring your entire cohesive team to the physical facility. Few large clinics do this, although I have seen it done effectively for small outreach clinics where a visiting specialist brings their own nurses, aides, and equipment.

Parallel Processing Model

Outpatient clinics using a parallel processing model reside in most smaller hospitals or private offices. These clinics may only have five to ten rooms and one to two nurses or aides. A solo receptionist checks in the patients and is aware of the office flow and can update patients and family members about any delays or issues. They can ensure that the patient has the needed paperwork, records, and testing before being placed in a room. Staff working in clinics with this model service only one specialty. They are trained in that specialty and are familiar with the needs of that specialty's physicians and other providers.

A physician in this clinic can easily have several patients in multiple rooms, work interactively with an advanced practitioner, and direct the nursing staff to perform in-office testing as needed. For example, the advanced practitioner could get the initial history, then have the nurse or aide get an electrocardiogram and perform a six-minute walk test. The physician could then see the patient and ask for an echo. In an advanced practice, the echo might be done down the hall at the same visit, followed by a wrap-up discussion with the physician and education with the nurses about recommended medication changes or next steps.

Parallel processing means that multiple patients are being seen at the same time and being attended to by multiple team members. Patients with unusually difficult issues do not stop the clinic flow. There is room for them to remain in the clinic while the issues are sorted out. This could be as simple as calling a nursing home or the pharmacy to ensure a proper medication reconciliation for an elderly patient with twenty listed prescriptions. Or it could be having the time to arrange for urgent inpatient admission without sending the patient through the emergency department first.

While I have worked in both models, I believe I took better care of the patients, saw more of them, and provided more comprehensive evaluations in the small clinic setting. In one outreach clinic, I did this with four rooms, an advanced practitioner, and one licensed practical nurse. We were able to effectively team. We knew the pattern, and the flow was effortless. Ancillary testing, including treadmill exercise testing, could be worked into the schedule. Between the three of us, we could accommodate urgent visits and adapt for late-arriving patients. One of our patients took three bus lines to get to the clinic. Not only did we fit him in, but we got him out in time to catch the last bus back home at the end of the day! We broke for lunch every day and finished on time every day. During the one-hour drive home, I felt satisfied, not exhausted or frustrated. The advanced practitioner carpooled with me, and we enjoyed the drives, developing a lasting friendship.

Unique Situations

Medicare Advantage

I recently explored a large Medicare Advantage plan offering value-based outpatient care. In this setting, the physicians are free to operate in whatever way they desire to deliver optimal patient care. Their clinics typically have ancillary testing readily available on-site, including blood testing, X-ray, and echocardiographic services. There is a limited pharmacy on-site for the most common medications so patients can leave the visit with what they need. Many older patients have limited ability to drive or otherwise get to a pharmacy. Having the ability to fill prescriptions on-site markedly improves compliance. Various support personnel are present, including therapists, social and caseworkers, dietitians, and educators. Providers in these models see patients more frequently (about once a month) and for longer visit times than the typical ten minutes found in many primary care practices. Patients enjoy the one-stop-shopping approach.

In this model, I've noticed there is a great ability to team well. The entire team is very effective at promoting a common goal and desire to provide comprehensive outpatient care to avoid costly inpatient admissions. Being co-located, providers can easily confer with pharmacists, therapists, social workers, and nurses to create and monitor patient care plans. Not only do patients get good care, the attention to prevention and follow-up yields large cost savings for Medicare. These types of plans are growing rapidly and are now found in many large cities. Providers are well compensated but not based on productivity. They are evaluated for quality and care metrics.

This model also allows the freedom to develop unique preventive approaches. For example, in one system, screening cardiac echocardiography is being used to find patients at risk for congestive heart failure. These echocardiograms would not be billable in a typical insurance model. While this approach is for patients using Medicare, ages sixty-five and up, I believe a similar approach could be easily implemented for our patients younger than sixty-five years of age.

Emergency and Twenty-Four-Hour Urgent Care
The emergency model has vastly different goals than an inpatient model, which is to identify and stabilize life-threatening issues. The structure of the team has a huge influence on its success. Structure is imperative to run efficiently and effectively, as seconds matter. They follow a team approach where the emergency department physician is the team leader *(captain)*, with nurses and aides under the team captain's direction. They also have a support team in the laboratory, X-ray, and housekeeping designed for their specific needs. For specialized illnesses, additional support teams have been established to assist the team captain. Most hospitals have a trauma team, a stroke team, and a heart attack team. These highly trained, protocol-driven teams are organized to provide the most effective patient care in the least amount of time, the *common goal.* These specialized protocols ensure

consistency based on best practice guidelines. Emergency-based teams constantly evaluate their progress, incorporate new processes, and tweak their performance to ensure that patient care is always optimized. They are the best template I've seen for effective teams.

Outside Factors

Of course, factors besides the practice environment influence how the team works. In academic settings, resident work-hour rules are one factor. There are defined rules limiting how many patients each resident can care for and how long each day they can provide care, which has significantly impacted continuity. While developed with good intent, there have been unintended consequences—additionally, the focus in many programs used to be on service rather than education. Residents were a cost-effective way to provide coverage for inpatient services and were expected to learn from experience and each other, with the senior residents mentoring the junior residents. It was not until the early 1980s that responsibility for patient care began to shift to the staff attending physicians. Before that, the attendings were there for support and teaching. We have moved into a stage where the staff attending physicians effectively have to care for and document in the EMR for each patient while also trying to provide education. I feel that this shift in focus has greatly hampered resident education. By removing the residents from the role of the primary caregiver, the pressure to learn and grow has been lessened.

While I do not suggest returning to the grueling hours I worked as a resident, I do believe we need to require and teach personal responsibility and critical thinking skills to our residents. Rather than having a group mentality of getting the work done, they need to be responsible for specific patients and expected to be functioning as the primary caregiver. Isn't the point for them to be equipped to be independent when they graduate? How else besides hands-on experience will they get it? They need to be prepared to be a team leader when they graduate!

Another factor that influences how teams work together is the varied shift schedules (eight-hour, twelve-hour) and hours of facility operation. As I mentioned above, it is possible to maintain effective teams if a premium on continuity is incorporated into staff shift scheduling. A consistent unit nurse manager and patient-nurse assignments will meet the key elements. Hours of operation will also influence teams. Running a team-based outpatient clinic during weekdays is fairly straightforward. Running a twenty-four-hour emergency room or urgent care clinic is a bit different, as discussed above.

Specific Implementation Tips

Academic Centers

- *Inpatient Services.* Design rotations to be a minimum of four weeks long. Coordinate residents and fellows to follow the same four-week pattern. Assign only three or four on-call attending physicians for the entire four weeks. Ensure a warm handoff every evening. Start morning rounds at the same time daily. Keep the resident physician the same for each patient. Preferably, the resident who admitted the patient would keep them. Keep the nursing assignments the same for each patient. Have daily multidisciplinary rounds, including ancillary services. Include the patient's nurse and the charge nurse in each patient's daily discussion and evaluation. Have a team debrief and discussion for all unexpected events or patient deaths. Celebrate patient successes as a team.
- *Outpatient Services.* Assign residents and fellows to specific staff supervisors (if applicable). Assign specific nurses to specific providers. Assign specific discharge clerks for specific providers. Train the clinic nurses in the specialty unique to their provider. Establish team routines, including protocols for in-office testing and typical follow-up instructions.

Community Hospitals

- *Inpatient Services.* Assign a charge nurse who is the same daily and is not caring for patients. Assign the same ancillary personnel to each specific unit. Keep the nursing assignments the same for each patient. Have daily multidisciplinary rounds, including ancillary services. Include the patient's nurse and the charge nurse in each patient's daily discussion and evaluation. Have a team debrief and discussion for all unexpected events or patient deaths. Celebrate patient successes as a team.

- *Office/Clinic.* Assign specific nurses to specific providers. Assign specific discharge clerks for specific providers. Establish team routines, including protocols, for in-office testing and typical follow-up instructions.

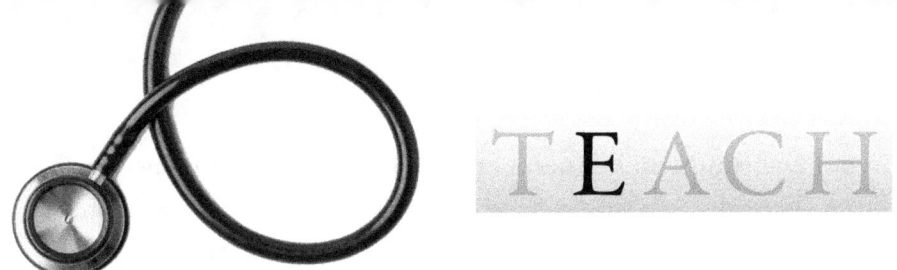

TEACH

Chapter 5

Encouraging Equity

I was sixteen when I built my first car. That's right, built. I spent my weekends at the junkyard (I think they are now called recycling centers) looking for the parts I needed—a rear window from a Mustang hatchback, the transmission from a Volkswagen, etc. The fiberglass kit I bought came with a full list of the additional needed items. I remember my excitement when that beautiful sky-blue car body was unloaded from the delivery truck. All my friends were drooling. Every night after finishing my homework, I worked in the garage, slowly but surely building that car. Nothing could keep me from my car. With grease on my hands, I watched a ten-inch black-and-white portable television propped on the chassis as I experienced the 1969 moon landing. Building *my* car, watching *my* astronauts land on the moon—it was a great evening!

The definition I am using for the term *equity* is ownership. Investors understand this concept, as do most homeowners. Your equity is your personal stake in a company, car, or home. We are invested in these things, and not just monetarily. Most of us long to own something. It could be physical, emotional, or psychological, but we desire a sense of ownership. Healthcare providers are no different. We work hard to care for our patients, make our office run well, or assist with efficient hospital care delivery. We even use the possessive when we talk: "my patients," "my office," "my hospital." But to have equity, we need to be acknowledged by the other persons working in our environment. We need a tangible "certificate of ownership," not unlike what we would have if we owned stock in Ford Motor Company. Of course, in the healthcare environment, this is typically not actual financial ownership, but it should be clear that we have either an emotional, physical, or positional stake in the system in which we operate. If we feel no equity—no ownership—in the system, we will not likely be engaged in a meaningful way. If we do not feel any sense of ownership with our patients, staff, or institution, we are just hired hands passing through.

Equity with Patients

With few exceptions, the modern delivery system has eliminated the sense of personal equity for providers. Do you feel like you have any equity in your patients, office, or hospital? Why is this even important? Because patient "ownership" is important for continuity of care. The provider is the patient's care captain and advocate. You build personal bonds and encourage each other. Patients want to feel known. Continuity achieves this and confirms that your practice of medicine makes a difference when you know how a patient is doing.

But many times, patients are seen in a clinic where any one of many providers could be assigned to them on that particular day. Scheduling priority may not be given to ensure they are always assigned to see you for follow-up. Instead, filling empty provider visit slots may be prioritized, which breaks the continuity of care. At a hospital where I recently worked, we could easily order a follow-up visit for patients we attended in the hospital. There was a convenient checkbox to indicate who the follow-up was to be with. Unfortunately, the intended provider was often overlooked when this electronic request was farmed out to any one of the fifteen scheduling staff (remember the team problem).

> Patients want to feel known. Continuity achieves this and confirms that your practice of medicine makes a difference when you know how a patient is doing.

Thus, "my patient" was scheduled to see my partner. Imagine how I feel when working in the clinic and realize my patient is in the office but not seeing me! It's disappointing and frustrating.

Many organizations have instituted a system of a primary provider; however, for patients with complex, specialty problems, their specialty care is often anything but consistent. Do you get frustrated when a patient you have seen weekly to manage a chronic condition (i.e., "your patient") is admitted to the hospital for an acute relapse, and *no one* calls you? Early in my career, I performed a cardiac catheterization on a patient "belonging to" a local internist. I did not inform the internist of this, and I got an earful from him the next day when the family had asked about the procedure he had no knowledge of! I never did that again.

Current practice is to use the EMR as a communication tool, effectively isolating providers from each other. Unfortunately, the EMR cannot communicate the nuances involved with some patients. I recently had trouble understanding why a patient I was consulting with seemed so difficult to keep stable. I called her primary care physician, and after a short discussion, it became abundantly clear why there was a problem. Her social situation (poorly described in the EMR) was complex and troublesome. Years of caring for her allowed her primary care physician to give information and insight that none of us had. She was "his patient," and his prolonged experience added invaluably to her care!

In the late 1980s, I treated a patient with an inferior heart attack. We opened his occluded artery, and he did so well that he was ready to go home by the third day. Unfortunately, he returned two days later with a serious complication—he had developed an acute ventricular septal defect, a hole in his heart muscle. Emergency surgery was required, and after twelve hours, he was brought back to his room with very low blood pressure and warnings that he was unlikely to survive. I joined the family in prayer that morning, and miraculously he improved.

After six weeks of treatment for many complications, he was well enough to go home. The man who left was not the same one who had presented to the emergency room six weeks earlier. He shared with me that he felt "different" about everything—the sun was brighter, his family more dear, and his pet dog and home were comforts. I had the privilege of caring for him for about another year, after which he died from complications of continued right heart failure. I loved seeing him and his family. We had a special bond that going through trials together can bring. He was always positive, even though his poor physical condition required that he be in a wheelchair, and he always had an encouraging word for the other patients. After he died, his daughter asked me something I had never been asked before or since. She asked me to give the eulogy at his funeral. I was honored and, of course, accepted. I drove to his hometown one day after work and stood before about fifty of his friends and family. I was sure that he had been kept alive for that additional year so he could impact others. He had certainly impacted me. He was "my patient," and I was committed to him and his family.

One of my patients was a woman I met in the middle of the night during her code blue. I was actually on call at home, and the resident phoned me to assist with her care. The house staff was performing cardiopulmonary resuscitation (CPR). Blood pressures were unobtainable in her arms, and she was on high doses of vasopressors. The situation sounded hopeless, but I drove in, and much to my surprise, when I felt the pulse in her leg, it was bounding. Her actual blood pressure was very high. Because of extensive narrowing in her subclavian arteries, the blood pressure in her arms was low, and many doctors had misdiagnosed her, ultimately stopping her antihypertensive medications and prescribing salt tablets.

My patient, Connie, underwent many interventional procedures after that. She was frequently readmitted with acute pulmonary edema since most caregivers did not accurately monitor her blood pressure to adjust her medications. Often, she would be taken to an outlying hospital where they did not know her. She was typically too sick to ask them to call me. Eventually, her daughter would call me, and we would have her transferred back to our hospital to treat her. We developed a special bond through these episodes. I recall that she was in our intensive care unit on a ventilator one time. When I visited, her eyes lit up as I entered, and we met halfway over the bed rail for a long hug. Connie was Catholic. I held her hand with her rosary between our palms and explained the test she was about to undergo. She always had that rosary. She always smiled (yes, even on the ventilator), and she was always positive about life. It kept her going. Against all odds, her positive attitude kept her going far longer than her physical condition warranted. It was an inspiration to me and to those who cared for her. The nurses were so sad when she died. They loved caring for her. She was always interested in their problems and concerned about their families. Not only was she "my patient," but she was "their patient" too.

I've chosen to foster a sense of equity for my patients by printing my personal phone number on my business cards for the past twenty years that I have owned a cell phone. (I realize many of you who are younger may not remember the days before cell phones.) I have only been called perhaps four times. In each case, it was appropriate, and I provided the needed advice without inconvenience to either of us. Once, I was called by an elderly woman's daughter to thank me for the intervention I had performed two years earlier and to let me know that her mom was still running around playing with the grandkids! I was having a busy day when I got the call, but knowing that "my patient" was doing well and appreciative made it worthwhile.

Equity with Offices

In days past, most physicians worked in small offices. They were *their* offices. They often owned the building, and their name was emblazoned on the door. When the phone was answered, it was announced: "Dr. Ahmed's office." In some cases, physicians worked out of the first floor of their homes. Everyone in town knew where Dr. Ahmed's office was. Due to many factors, owning a private office in the current healthcare system has become financially impractical.

Practices have been purchased and integrated into multispecialty clinics. Accelerated by the Affordable Care Act, accountable care organizations have become the norm, with outpatient and inpatient services controlled by large systems. Providers now work in hospital-owned shared spaces. We may work in multiple shared spaces, doing outreach clinics or covering multiple hospitals each week. We share rooms. We share computers. We share staff. We don't own anything, and when we leave for the day, it will all be turned over to someone else in the morning. This makes teaming difficult, as discussed in the first chapter, but it also reduces the sense of equity. What if I wanted a picture of my family on my desk at work? How about a display of my diplomas or a favorite piece of artwork? Where would I put it? I have no equity in my work environment. I am just a worker moving from one shared space to another. When the phone is answered at my space for the day, it is announced: "Cardiology." It is no longer our office, just a place where some cardiology care is delivered on that day. On its own, this does not seem like a big deal, but it is the sum of many small changes that have led to the sense of isolation felt by so many providers.

Equity with Hospitals

I have privileges at many hospitals. This is not by choice. If I had my way, I would practice at one facility all the time. But the days when I can say "this is my hospital" are over for many of us, particularly in academic practice in large cities. Many of us now practice at several hospitals, partly due to system aggregation and partly due to insurance requirements. And if one hospital (or system) is struggling, I can always move to another. I can easily pit them against each other.

I was involved in one city where groups of physicians had privileges at multiple hospitals and would use their patient volume to influence what they wanted to be done for them at each facility. There was no loyalty, no sense of ownership in the hospital, and no sense of partnership in a shared vision. Such a lack of equity leads to perverted goals and fuels an environment of mistrust, discontent, and conflict. I have also had the privilege of working in a system that, by charter, must be led by a physician. Of course, such systems are still concerned about business and billing, but I believe there is a subtle difference when it comes to provider concerns. Providers run the administration, and, despite being out of daily patient care activities, they still have a better understanding of our needs. Some of the most well-respected systems were started by physicians and are still governed by physicians: Mayo Clinic, Cleveland Clinic, Geisinger Health System, Lahey Clinic, and Sanger Clinic, to name a few. Each of these was undoubtedly felt to be "my hospital" by the founding providers!

Conversely, I don't often hear hospital administrators saying, "Dr. Cater is our cardiologist." Unfortunately, as noted above, we may contribute to this issue by splitting our loyalties and attention among different systems. Administrators are afraid to institute changes that may be perceived as favoring one group over another group. After all, what would happen to the bottom line if the group who feels slighted were to take their patients elsewhere? This is not an easy problem to solve. I once tried to broker a win-win situation for multiple private groups to join a hospital system effort to create a world-class service line. After three years of effort, we could not find a situation that would satisfy each of the stakeholders. In my opinion, this was the direct result of a years-long decline in trust and alignment between the hospital and the providers.

In some cases, moving toward a better sense of equity will require significant realignment. However, I still believe the ultimate benefits of a healthy equity relationship will be worth the effort.

Steps You Can Take

Make every effort to assign each patient to a unique and consistent physician, both for primary care and specialty care.
Most current EMR systems have ways to track this, but it may require some higher-level programming and attention to accomplish it.

Develop an easy, efficient system for communication among the patient's provider team.

While many EMRs will forward notes to other providers, it is hard to have a simple communication similar to the personal text messaging we have all become used to. Again, many EMRs have messaging functions, but they are not easily accessible, and the culture does not encourage their use. This can be changed, but it will require a top-down approach.

Ensure the patient understands who their provider is and how to get hold of them.

Give out business cards with direct contact numbers. As I noted, I have had my personal cell phone printed on my business card for years. It has never been abused. Encourage the use of patient portal systems. Reward patients for using them by attending promptly to their requests. My personal family's experience is that portal requests are often ignored until a phone call is made requesting some attention. This defeats the purpose!

Make it easy for patients to find their provider information on the system website.

I have yet to find a hospital website that has an easy way to find provider contact information. You can search by specialty, but rarely by location or address. If you do find the listing, you will likely be directed to a central scheduling number and not the actual office.

Encourage community and communication between providers by making it easy to contact each other.

We all have direct lines, or back lines to our offices. Why do we hide these from each other? Spend some time developing an effective provider directory for us to use: list back lines, assistant lines, cell phones, etc. How can we complain about not being contacted about our patients if we make it so hard to find us?

Provide a primary office space for each provider.
Allow the provider to decorate it and make it their own. If two providers need to share one space, try to provide two desks so that at least the desk can be personalized. I like to keep some reference materials nearby; providing a space to store these makes me feel like my work effort is important.

Display the provider's name at the office, on the letterhead, and on patient communications.
There is no excuse for not having signs. They can be made for a few dollars at any office supply store. Similarly, letterhead need not be bought in bulk. It can be printed out as needed given the correct template. My current medical assistant has created signs for us; granted, they are handwritten on copy paper with double-sided tape, but I appreciate the effort!

When a call is answered, identify the office by the provider's name.
Create the bond with patients by answering calls as "Dr. Jones's office," even if it is only for the day!

Identify practitioners within the hospital.
Develop easy-to-find personal mechanisms to contact them. There is no excuse for any staff member to be unable to contact us. These tools should be simple and fast.

Provide an easy way to see which providers are in the hospital that day or which providers are providing new consult services for the day.
Ensure that the contact method for each provider is up to date. In one of my current hospitals, after at least ten calls to the operator to request a change, I am still contacted by my personal cell phone rather than the hospital cell phone. I don't mind getting a call on my personal phone, but I don't always carry it with me, and many areas of the hospital don't get service.

Things to Avoid

Avoid running clinics that pair patients with a pool of providers.
Both patients and their families need a consistent provider they can develop a relationship with. Even though I currently work only every other week, my patients are assigned to see me, not my partner provider covering the alternate weeks.

Don't forget to communicate with your colleagues if you consult on, admit, or otherwise interact with one of their established patients.
Again, having an easy method can facilitate this communication and establish a new cultural norm.

Don't assign patients to a "team."
This devalues the patient and the provider. Team A will not be caring for them; Dr. Manheim will! Assigning personal connections will foster improved care and attention for that patient. Someone assigned to nothing will attend to nothing.

Don't assign providers to a cubicle for the day.
Please give them a personal space to use. Often, the dirty utility room is assigned more space!

Avoid rotating practitioners among practice locations.
If multiple hospitals need coverage, assign specific providers to specific hospitals. If that is not possible, at the very least, provide consistent coverage for several days at a time. Most patients have a hospital stay of two to four days. Why, then, do we change providers daily?

Don't call providers by their specialty within the hospital.
We should never hear "Call Cardiology." When we answer the phone, we should not be asked if we are Cardiology! I am not Cardiology. Cardiology is the study of the heart and vascular system. I am a person, and I have a name.

Specific Implementation Tips

Academic Centers

- *Inpatient Services.* Assign each patient a primary resident and a primary attending physician. Make sure this is clear to the patient. Process all decisions and care changes through these constant providers. During evenings away from the hospital, ensure that the providers covering are aware of who the primary providers are and understand that the covering providers are to provide a status report the next day to the primary providers. Keep the primary nursing assignment the same for each patient, so the patient has a consistent advocate. Ensure that any unexpected or unusual events are communicated to the primary providers in a timely fashion. Ensure that the primary provider gives the hospital follow-up, rather than a transition-of-care team person who has never interacted with the patient. Ensure that the patient knows how to contact their primary provider. If the patient no longer needs a particular provider's care, ensure a clearly communicated process of transferring primary responsibility to a new provider. This process especially applies to specialty care where close follow-up may be provided by the specialist for a period of time after hospitalization but then can be transferred to a generalist for long-term care.
- *Outpatient Services.* List providers by name in your office building. Make sure it is clear where a patient would go to find that provider or their staff. Ensure that volunteers, who are often placed around large complexes to assist patients, have clear reference materials to specifically locate individual providers by name. Assign patients to specific individual providers, not a pool of teammates. Assign specific nurses to specific providers. Ensure that the patient has a clear mechanism for contacting their provider, either with a direct office line or an easy-to-use digital chart interface. When patients do use the digital interface, ensure that providers (or their staff) are monitoring and respond in a

timely fashion. Ensure your digital interface or public website has an easily identifiable mechanism for a user to find and contact specific named providers.

Community Hospitals

- *Inpatient Services.* Ensure that the operator and each patient care area have a listing of all active providers and a mechanism to contact them. Attempt to make this contact method similar for all rather than a pager for one, a cell phone for another, and an EMR message for yet another. Encourage persons with questions or concerns about a specific patient to contact the provider directly rather than have a unit clerk relay a message. Foster events or meetings that allow providers to mingle with and get to know their colleagues.
- *Office/Clinic:* Establish fixed office locations for specific providers. Label them accordingly. Ensure an up-to-date clinic building directory with office locations and specific provider names. Phones in each office should be answered with the physician's name.

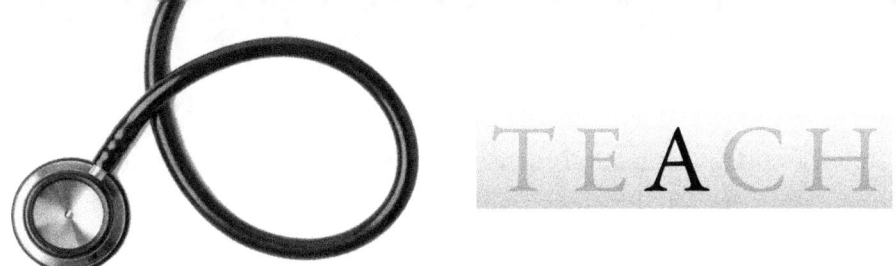

TEACH

Chapter 6

Involving Providers in Administrative Functions

D r. Barnes was working to fix something again. Three of us from the catheterization lab were asked to be part of a task force, as she called it. We groaned. This probably meant more work, as if we didn't have enough to do! But Doc had noticed that our turnaround time between cases was higher than she liked. Mr. Nelson from the corporate office suggested that perhaps we needed to work longer hours to fit in the number of cases required by our budget. Thankfully, Doc disagreed. At the first task force meeting, she told us that she believed we could figure out a solution. She was confident that we could manage our own workflow to be efficient *and* get home on time. It was difficult to understand what we could do at first, but with her encouragement, we started digging into the problem. Doc was right! By implementing a few changes in the way we staffed our lab and assigned the patients, we reduced our turnaround time from forty minutes to only eighteen. After that, we had a new appreciation for Dr. Barnes. She was pretty good *outside* the lab too! Better yet, she understood our issues and believed in our capabilities.

The word *administration* has gotten a bad reputation among physicians. We immediately think of the hospital or clinic business leaders with whom we don't get along very well. This is unfortunate. Let me be clear; I am not using *administration* as a synonym for clerical

83

activities. I am using *administration* to describe the important business and operational issues that impact our practice settings. In my opinion, the assignment of, and concentration of, all administrative duties within the organization's business leaders is one of the reasons providers are not thriving. While few are formally trained in business and finance, providers like Dr. Barnes all like to be involved in process management and developing procedures that improve their ability and satisfaction in providing patient care. As noted in chapter 5, many of the great institutions were founded and led by physician administrators. Their entire structure was designed, tweaked, and nurtured by physician leaders. To be fair, many current providers are not interested in administration as it presently exists. But even just a few years ago, when physicians owned their personal practice, they were empowered administrators. They set the office's goals, the expectations for employee behavior, and the bar for patient care to be delivered there. Now, they are typically just employees in a provider cost center. Outside of the medical staff group membership, current providers have little if any input into the administrative workings of their practice environment.

Administrative Explosion!

The hiring of hospital administrators has grown 3,200 percent between 1975 and 2010, while physician growth has only been 150 percent over the same period, similar to population growth.[8] Clearly, something has changed! Several major healthcare-related governmental or billing policy changes affected the growth of administrator positions. Among them were RVU-based billing, diagnosis related group (DRG) hospital payments, and the 1996 Health Insurance Portability and Accountability Act (HIPAA).

My personal recollection of this time period was one of increasing movement to EMR-based documentation and increased emphasis on billing activities. As I mentioned previously, I was in academic practice at that time and was afforded two to three days per week of protected time. During that time, I supervised three research nurses and two research fellows, as well as an animal technician and an active animal investigation laboratory. Our team was very productive in producing abstracts and manuscripts; we attended several national and international meetings each year to present our work.

Also, during that time, there was a shift from the institution (hospital or medical school/university) supporting my salary. Whereas our team's activity was considered part of the overall mission (and included in the general budget), it became evident that any academic (non-billable) activity would require alternative funding. So the highly integrated clinical-research team became split. The hospital-employed nurses in the catheterization lab were no longer allowed to assist with any research-related activity that might be carried out in the lab. Research-employed nurses would have to come in to complete that paperwork. If I wanted to work two days in the research labs, I would need to find two days' worth of outside funding for my salary. The days of the clinician-scientist were coming to an end. It became increasingly difficult to excel at both, especially since principal investigator salary funding was generally excluded from external grants.

Some of us were able to continue clinical investigation by using evening and weekend hours for any non-billing activity. How this relates to the rise in administrator hiring is not entirely clear to me. Still, there was a clear shift from being allowed to use my skills and energy to advance the academic mission to being required to earn my keep by focusing on billing activities. Of course, billing activities require an enormous number of administrators to manage the myriad of different contracts and documentation requirements.

The Division between Providers and Administrators

Fast forward to the present. A recent study in a large academic system comparing providers to administrators found that "the majority (90 percent) of participants described difficulties connecting and collaborating with members of other professional groups. Perceived issues involved recent changes that were well-intended from an organizational care perspective but complicated physicians' workflows and abilities to engage in academic activities."[9] At some point during the past twenty years, providers and administrators have become disconnected at best and adversarial in many cases.

Dr. Kealy Ham, a pulmonologist who has begun working in administration, believes that physicians may feel they're being told how to do their jobs by people who have never done their jobs. At the same time, administrators looking at the finances feel the need to work toward better efficiency to reduce costs.[10] I agree with her and share several recent examples of this disconnect below.

> While there are new regulatory, oversight, and financial complexities, they do not justify the near-total exclusion of providers from the administrative function of the system.

A host of factors have eroded provider involvement in administration. Most importantly, as discussed in chapter 5, providers no longer have equity in their environment. Further, they believe the business "experts" think they lack the requisite training or common sense to manage a complex delivery system appropriately. While there are new regulatory, oversight, and financial complexities, they do not justify the near-total exclusion of providers from the administrative function of the system. Finally, providers are felt to be most effective (read *profitable*) if they are focused on billable activities. While this is logical, it ignores the human and emotional side of practicing medicine.

Reengaging Providers in the Operation of Healthcare Systems

Providers are not machines. We are not immune to the pain and suffering we attend to day in and day out. I think most of us would appreciate having some say in our practice environment and some breaks from the action to regroup and deal with our colleagues rather than just patients. Practicing medicine is an art requiring flexibility, creativity, and resilience. It is not an assembly line where we just push the buttons mindlessly to generate CPT codes! Building in some administrative activity is a way to recognize the wisdom and knowledge of providers.

It makes them feel like part of the team and engenders a sense of equity in the system. I felt this way in the early 1990s when I was overseeing a team of nearly twenty clinical catheterization lab and interventional research staff. It is hard to feel much like part of something larger if the only metrics I am judged by are my RVUs and how rapidly I complete my EMR charting so that the bill can be "dropped."

Involving providers in administrative activities must be genuine, however. I once worked in a for-profit hospital system. We were in the process of replacing our X-ray suite, and the hospital enlisted me (a cardiologist) and the directors of two other departments who used the suite, vascular surgery and interventional radiology, to review potential replacements. We were told that the hospital system had a favorable pricing contract with one vendor, but during direct questioning, they consistently told us that we could make the final decision on vendor selection. The system offered by the preferred vendor had several features that made it nearly unusable for some common radiology and surgical applications. We unanimously chose a different vendor that did not have these limitations and made our recommendations. You can imagine our disappointment when we learned that, in fact, the preferred vendor was the only option and that our opinion was not going to be honored. Hours of meetings, site visits, and discussions between three department directors were wasted. Instead of being included for our expertise (after all, we were the ones who had to use the system to treat patients), we were led on and then dishonored.

In contrast to this experience, I was given a chance in a different hospital to select an X-ray vendor for two new suites (of note, in 1990.) I was part of an administrative team

> Practicing medicine is an art requiring flexibility, creativity, and resilience. It is not an assembly line where we just push the buttons mindlessly to generate CPT codes! Building in some administrative activity is a way to recognize the wisdom and knowledge of providers.

including facilities, biomedical engineering, and architectural design specialists. We worked together, each bringing our unique expertise to the discussion. We chose to go with a vendor who wanted to break into our market and place two state-of-the-art systems to be used as a show site for prospective customers. We were able to design very functional and aesthetically pleasing spaces. The attention we received from the vendor and visiting colleagues was a big win for the institution.

Models for Effective Collaboration

I want to be very clear that I respect the expertise and hard work that my administrative business colleagues provide. I have been fortunate to work alongside many who have welcomed my input and shared administrative duties with me. I participated in a dyad structure while working at a large, physician-led health system. Each physician leader was paired with a business leader. We were jointly responsible for the operational and financial aspects of the service line. We each brought unique perspectives to the issues that arose and potential solutions. My knowledge of patient care and physician attitudes complemented their operational and financial background. Together we navigated some uncertain times in the medical care environment, including the initiation of the 2010 Affordable Care Act. We grew the business and improved care delivery and patient outcomes.

By working together and including many frontline physician leaders, we actually built a new heart hospital during a time when many systems were canceling projects. We got very intentional and critical of the initial design parameters (specified by a consulting firm). We reduced the number of clinic rooms in the main hospital, recognizing the shift to outreach sites, and combined overlapping services into common areas (vascular ultrasound and cardiac echo). We also designed all inpatient beds to be "swing beds," capable of serving as an unmonitored room up to a fully equipped critical care bed. Patients never had to change rooms, as the level of care they received adjusted instead. In this critical process, we freed up an entire floor of the new building, enabling another service line to remain on campus and saving a million dollars. Both clinicians and administrators were happy with the end product, and it came in under budget! Unfortunately, most of my colleagues have never been afforded this degree of involvement.

Typically, physicians are asked by the administration to fulfill only those tasks that are required by the regulatory or oversight bodies. Depending on State or Joint Commission on Accreditation of Healthcare Organizations (JCAHO) guidelines, providers may be required to be directors of certain hospital services. In Ohio, this is required for cardiac catheterization laboratories in smaller hospitals. Unfortunately, physicians assigned to these director roles are often in name only with no actual authority or influence. Authority is assumed by others in the organization. In some instances, the hospital has to pay significant sums to entice a physician to fulfill this role in which they have no actual responsibilities! How different might it be if the physician actually had some influence over the administrative duties of such a position? They might feel like part of the team, like they have some equity in the system!

Alternative Forms of Involvement for Providers

Of course, providers have abused the director positions as well. At one hospital where I worked, I was one of only a few employed physicians. There was no medical school in this city and very little academic influence over the care delivered. When I arrived, the hospital was paying over twelve million dollars yearly in director fees! Providers had been abusing these positions, sometimes holding directorships at three or four different hospitals. While not explicitly stated, the implication was that a hospital might be favored for admissions if they assigned directorships (with huge stipends) to providers in certain groups. This type of arrangement gives the administration a sour taste for providers and does a disservice to those providers who would like to be involved and provide input and expertise to administrative activities.

At one point in my career, I explored medical system consulting. I applied and interviewed at several prominent consulting firms. Unfortunately, these firms are run almost entirely by business professionals. They had no idea how a physician could add value to their services even though their services were often contracted to assist hospitals with physician problems. These firms consisting of business professionals are highly sought out (and highly paid) by the business professionals who administer the healthcare delivery systems. And these business professionals are trying to figure out how to profitably administer patient care, which they have never provided, while effectively excluding all input from the providers who do it day in and day out! Many of these firms are run similarly to legal practices. The partners are responsible for generating a book of business, and none felt that I could generate any new business for them. Apparently, in their experience, advice from a seasoned practitioner was of little value to their clients.

Examples of Successful Teaming on Administrative Efforts

The exclusion of providers from meaningful administrative oversight is to everyone's detriment. Providers can provide valuable insight and oversight if they are given the opportunity. At the request of engaged providers, one small hospital at which I worked established a CEO-physician leader forum. We met quarterly over a casual dinner to discuss issues of concern to the providers and to be updated on administrative issues. Any issues we identified were tracked on a dashboard, and many important system improvements resulted from this collaborative effort. So I know it can work, but it will take dedicated effort and protected time to accomplish.

On a related but slightly different note, I have also assisted with several experiential programs for non-clinicians. These were designed to help them fully understand providers' day-to-day needs and experiences. We developed a week-long immersion program for sales personnel in a very forward-thinking program organized and supported by an industry manufacturer of cardiology equipment. Sales members were partnered with busy providers. They came to the hospital when we did; they were by our side all day and ate (or not) when we did. They carried a pager at night, and they came in when we were called in. After a week, every participant remarked that they had no idea what our days were like! Their eyes were opened, and they felt much more capable of interacting with and understanding us. Years later, many sought me out to comment on how life-changing the experience was. It would be very easy for hospital administrators to experience the same thing; it would be a week well spent.

In a different system, we organized a daylong shadow event for existing and prospective donors to the hospital foundation. Again, they got to see what we did and the issues we faced. They experienced firsthand how the space or equipment they contributed to facilitated patient care. Not only did the experience benefit the non-clinicians, but the providers had a chance to break out of the daily routine and show pride in their work.

Steps You Can Take

Incorporate protected time for providers to participate in the administration of the system.
Providing protected time (or compensated time for nonemployees) for these duties indicates that they are valued and important to the system.

Give providers important tasks, not just regulatory necessities.
Examples might be leading a continuous quality improvement committee to reduce the length of stay for patients with congestive heart failure or overseeing the office staffing committee involved in hiring, firing, and evaluations. This is very different from the JCAHO-required committee meetings actually run by system administrators with figure-head physician involvement. Providers know the difference and would appreciate the chance to participate in meaningful activities.

Seek out provider input for major system decisions before the decision has been made.
Providers may be the last to hear that the system has just committed to purchasing the small struggling hospital ten miles away. What may

seem like a good business decision may wreak havoc on the provision of patient care, provider scheduling, call schedules, and the like.

Look in-house for advice before hiring outside consulting firms to tell us how to be better providers.

These outside firms will just tap into the internal solutions that have not been discovered yet! At the end of the day, the change will be implemented by the existing providers, not by the consultants. The same applies to hiring external "change management" specialists.

Develop provider-administrator discussion forums.

Adequately support them and actively work on the identified issues.

Design experiences for senior administrators or board members to shadow busy clinicians.

I had the pleasure to work with Dr. Ronald Paulus, who, when he was CEO of Mission Health in Asheville, NC, commented, "Board members who had been through an immersion day reported learning more about the organization in six hours of shadowing than in six years of board service."[11]

Things to Avoid

Don't assume providers have no business or process management abilities.

Many providers have successful and interesting outside lives. They own and run successful restaurants, farms, stores, rental properties, and small companies. Some are inventors, entrepreneurs, investors, and employers. They can bring these same skills to healthcare.

Don't assign providers to committees on which they have no responsibility or authority.
Figurehead appointments, especially ones that are compensated, are not only of little value to the system but may raise questions related to Stark Law violations.

Don't exclude providers from functional committees that govern day-to-day care delivery.
While multiple meetings may not be desirable, a well-organized meeting over dinner with good staff support can lead to meaningful change and build equity and loyalty.

Don't ask providers to participate in administrative activities if you have no intention of considering their advice seriously.
We don't want to be patronized.

Specific Implementation Tips

Academic Centers

- Most academic centers focus administrative tasks only on the department or division chairs. Instead, actively encourage younger providers to participate in administrative committees. Make this a priority, and build in time for it. Ensure that the committee is well run with minutes, agendas, and specifically assigned action items.
- There may be many seemingly minor decisions at department level to be made. Resist making these at the chair level and instead enlist a few younger providers to explore the possibilities and report back to the department with recommendations. If necessary, provide administrative support to this ad hoc committee, as many providers have never been trained in running meetings or producing deliverables.
- Administrators must be genuine if they include providers in administrative work. Be willing to listen and understand the

clinical or implementation concerns even if they seem at odds with traditional business management practice.

- Set up some standing committees for provider engagement and input, especially around the issues of EMR and patient flow. Ensure that these committees have an allocated budget that can be used to address suggestions. Typically, this involves support from the information technology personnel or paid consultation with the EMR provider. When meaningful ideas are brought up to enhance or improve the EMR, we are often told that there are no resources who can work on it or that it is not in the budget.
- Actively encourage provider participation in leadership development activities. Give protected time for these activities. Most large businesses, business schools, and some medical schools have such programs. These are different from patient engagement or patient satisfaction-oriented programs.
- Suggest and pay for several months of professional physician administrative coaching.

Community Hospitals

- Many functions run through the medical staff. Rarely, however, have I seen resources dedicated to support this body (other than a monthly dinner). Hospitals need to create a budget to support projects suggested by the medical staff committees.
- Create a rotation system for administrative committees so that multiple providers get the opportunity to participate.
- Encourage active participation by directors. They should be leading committee meetings, not a hospital staff person. Compensation should be directly tied to participation and contribution. Compensation must be fair market value for hourly billing.
- Develop physician-administration forums, and institute shadow days for administrators.

- Demonstrate your commitment to provider growth and future administrative input:
  - Sponsor leadership development courses for your key physicians.
  - Offer paid professional physician coaching (perhaps four to six sessions).

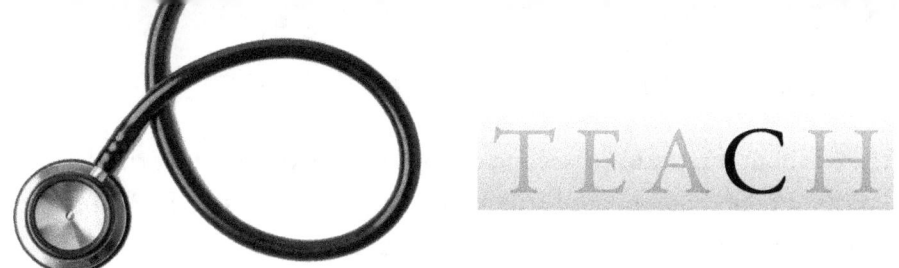

Chapter 7

Building Community for Connectedness

My experience over the past forty years has been a gradual shift away from activities that build and value community. Let me share again what it used to be like to have community. As discussed in chapter 2, when I was a cardiology fellow in the early 1980s, our section would meet every weekday at 7:00 a.m. for an all-inclusive conference. It was attended by the staff physicians, fellows, residents, and often our nurses or technicians. Each day was devoted to an interesting topic in one of five general areas. One day it might be ECG, another cardiac catheterization, etc. The fellows would often present a case study with a literature review. It was a wonderful time of learning together and a lively discussion between the mentors and the mentees. Over two years, we really got to know each other and understand our community values. Believe it or not, there were no doughnuts, no industry support, and no free breakfast! Yet everyone came and participated.

Building Daily Connections

When I was interviewing for a job in the 1980s, I traveled to a prominent physician-led clinic. The group had about twenty providers, including cardiologists and cardiothoracic surgeons. The group met daily at 7:00 a.m. for breakfast and discussed the day's activities. They talked about interesting cases and divided up the workload for the day. I did not take that job, but I still remember how impressed I was that this group of providers truly functioned as a community and looked out for each other! And I remain friends with one of the cardiologists who interviewed me there.

During the 1990s, I was fortunate to spend a year working in a heart hospital in Germany. We were very busy clinically; however, I remember well the daily breaks in the midmorning where we would stop and have a coffee and pretzel bread! We stopped for lunch every day and ate together in the dining room, me practicing my German and they their English. We took time to relax and connect despite often performing five to fifteen catheterizations or interventions per day in each of the three labs! I still feel a sense of community with that hospital and the colleagues I worked with there. Among the most important relationships was the administrative assistant to the hospital director. She ensured I had every need (including housing, a car, and schools for the kids) attended to and that I was integrated into the hospital activity.

In the early 2010s, I tried to institute a daily morning group meeting at a large teaching hospital. I was met with fairly staunch resistance. Many of the reasons given for not wanting such a time were quite valid. Patient care activities needed to start as soon as possible to get through the number of persons needing testing. Our days often stretched until 6:00 or 7:00 p.m., and getting back to work so early was felt to be stressful and not enjoyable. Further, due to multiple outreach programs, off-campus activities, and the like, at most, 50 to 60 percent of likely participants would be on campus on any given day. We were never able to institute a time to gather as a group, which in my estimation severely impaired our sense of community. The business of patient care consumed every minute of the day. There was no time for coffee breaks, no time for shared lunches, and participation in the mandatory conferences was spotty at best!

The overall community norm was to pack as much patient care activity into each day as possible. Despite my desire for our department to have time together, the ever-present expectation to do more kept the providers conflicted. They never felt comfortable or relaxed in a meeting or gathering, as there was always more work. Packing as much as possible into each day may be good for the bottom line, but it is shortsighted, and we are now all paying the price for overlooking community building. Provider burnout is rampant!

What Makes Up a Sense of Community?

In a seminal 1986 study, McMillan and Chavis identify four elements of a sense of community:

- Membership: the feeling of belonging or of sharing a sense of personal relatedness
- Influence: mattering, making a difference to a group, and of the group mattering to its members
- Reinforcement: integration and fulfillment of needs
- Shared emotional connection[12]

Tools such as the Sense of Community Index (SCI) and its brief form, the Brief Sense of Community Scale (BSCS), have been used to assess the four elements of sense of community noted by McMillan and Chavis.[13] Unfortunately, very little data exist using validated tools to measure the sense of community in healthcare systems (except for some long-term mental health units.) Nonetheless, it is easy to imagine that practicing in an environment where one feels like

> Packing as much as possible into each day may be good for the bottom line, but it is shortsighted, and we are now all paying the price for overlooking community building.

they belong, has emotional connections, and influences care delivery would improve practitioner well-being. While not typically discussed in terms of community, both nursing and hospital leaders understand some of the basic tenets. A recent editorial discussing common hospital administrative mistakes states:

Maintaining relationships with physicians is an integral component leading to a hospital's current and future financial success. "The only ones who admit patients and provide mainstream revenue to hospitals is the medical staff," says Joseph DeSilva, FACHE, partner at The Kiran Consortium Group, a healthcare advisory and professional services firm. ... Most of these common mistakes can be avoided simply by ensuring the physicians and the rest of the medical staff are appreciated, understood and heard.[14]

To me, that sounds a lot like ensuring that they feel part of the "community."

Dr. Kenneth Bertka, who leads physician integration at Catholic Health Partners in Toledo, Ohio, works with the Center for Creative Leadership to train leaders, including physician leaders, in a three-step process. The first step is establishing a direction—achieving a shared understanding of goals and strategy around a team approach. The second step is aligning people—removing traditional healthcare silos, sharing resources, and establishing new teams that lead to changes in existing roles. Finally, he suggests that creating an environment of trust, transparency, and mutual respect will fan the sparks of passion into steps of commitment (author's paraphrase).[15]

Notice that each of these steps helps to build a sense of community among the providers and their institutions.

Similar issues have been more extensively discussed in the nursing literature. Rose O. Sherman, EdD, RN, FAAN, is director of the Nursing Leadership Institute at the Christine E. Lynn College of Nursing, Florida Atlantic University. She writes, "We also know from nursing research that nurses have an innate need to feel connected and valued as members of a community. This sense of community must extend beyond the nursing staff to interdisciplinary team members and support staff who spend time on the unit. To deliver patient-centered care and improve patient satisfaction, every staff member must feel a unified commitment. That starts with a sense of belonging and ownership." She further states, "To build a strong community, everyone must feel like a valued member, including interdisciplinary team members and housekeeping and engineering staff."[16] Based on her other writings, I would argue that Shannon had no intention of excluding physicians and other providers from the community!

Building Community Still Exists in Some Places
Not all community-building activities have been lost, however. When I was at one large system with multiple hospitals and over fifty outpatient delivery sites, I experienced some powerful community-building activities. When challenged by upcoming government-mandated healthcare changes, we formed multidisciplinary teams to address focused aspects of our care delivery to streamline and eliminate waste while maximizing patient outcomes. These task forces often lasted up to a year. During our many meetings, we developed a sense of community with our team members and the overall institutional goals. In the area of heart failure management, we went even further. We joined with two other large health systems and worked on multisystem solutions to care for this chronic condition. Our community grew even larger, and we all benefited from the shared experiences.

In the same system, we also developed a sense of community in that our compensation was in part based on system-wide goals. The entire organization had three to four major goals each year. As discussed in chapter 2, accomplishing these goals required working in small task groups with many different inputs. These meetings fostered a sense of community as we worked together for over a year. And in the end, we had the satisfaction of accomplishing something together. Working together in teams is a great way to build community. Each member who has influence is working toward the same goal, the goal is well defined, and there is an expectation that the whole group will accomplish the goal.

I have also been very fortunate to have experienced community among my colleagues on the lecture circuit and members of the professional societies to which I belong. In these settings, we could take some time to relax, dine together, work on committees together, produce guidelines or position papers, and influence care delivery. Often away from home and (usually) away from patient care activities, we could relate as colleagues without the pressure to get back to work. My closest friendships were formed during these experiences. Unfortunately, few providers have this opportunity to interact with their peers on any regular basis. Thus, it is all the more important that we build community *within* the typical care delivery system. In the typical system, social gatherings are rare. I suspect I have been out for lunch or dinner with a colleague from my own institution fewer than twenty times over forty years. This is notably unlike my experience in Germany, where we were together almost daily. The closest thing to this I have experienced in the US is a monthly citywide case review session sponsored by a healthcare device company at a local restaurant. Unfortunately, many institutions actually prohibit participation in such community-building activities due to perceived inappropriate industry influence even though the meeting is organized and run by physicians with no commercial discussion.

Tools for Building a Sense of Community

Many well-functioning companies and communities exist as role models for addressing these concerns. The Gallup Organization has studied many organizations to determine what factors contribute to a healthy organization, where employees feel valued and are engaged. They have condensed the findings down to twelve key questions every organization must answer in order to increase productivity and profitability, reduce absenteeism, and increase loyalty to the company and the customer (our patients).[17] These key questions are detailed in table 3.

Q01. I know what is expected of me at work.

Q02. I have the materials and equipment I need to do my work right.

Q03. At work, I have the opportunity to do what I do best every day.

Q04. In the last seven days, I have received recognition or praise for doing good work.

Q05. My supervisor, or someone at work, seems to care about me as a person.

Q06. There is someone at work who encourages my development.

Q07. At work, my opinions seem to count.

Q08. The mission or purpose of my organization makes me feel my job is important.

Q09. My associates or fellow employees are committed to doing quality work.

Q10. I have a best friend at work.

Q11. In the last six months, someone at work has talked to me about my progress.

Q12. This last year, I have had opportunities at work to learn and grow.

Table 3. Gallup Q12 Questions

As you read through these, do you see some common threads? Employees want to feel empowered, appreciated, and supported. In other words, they want community. If they feel a sense of community, they are happier at work. The same is true for healthcare providers!

Linzer, et al., have studied provider trust in their organizations in varied primary care settings. They found that organizational loyalty, a safe culture, a sense of belonging, helping other providers in need, and the overall trustworthiness of the organization were important for developing strong individual provider trust.[18] They have developed tools that can assist in evaluating work-life balance and provide data to empower local quality improvement initiatives. The same group has proposed ten steps for preventing burnout in internal medicine, many of which are similar to those I discuss here.[19]

Compensation and Community Can Be Complementary

At the risk of touching the third rail, I want to discuss the financial incentives for maximizing work activities at the expense of community building. Provider compensation has always been more than adequate in my opinion. However, there has been increasing pressure to maintain or increase compensation levels. Many factors drive this. Among them are dramatic increases in education debt accumulated during provider education. After implementing RVU-based fee schedules, procedural activities became far more profitable than cognitive services.

Further, payments from Medicare and Medicaid have actually fallen, especially when adjusted for inflation. Finally, a host of unfunded mandates were added to the delivery system (e.g., EMR use, continuing medical education [CME] requirements, quality metrics, etc.). The unavoidable consequence of a payment system based on service provision using CPT codes is that it now requires more service provision to generate the same level of reimbursement. So if systems want more time for community building, they must reduce service provision per provider and, ultimately, provider compensation. Some providers, especially those without large debt, would gladly trade some compensation for a less hectic, more fulfilling day-to-day schedule. In the current system, this is untenable for most providers.

In the fourth chapter, I mentioned a Medicare Advantage plan that I interviewed with. I bring it up again here as it demonstrates the ability to build community and remain financially viable *at the same time.* You may wonder how they can maintain high compensation levels while enjoying more sense of community and a slower pace of care. The key is that their reimbursement is not tied to the provision of billable CPT services. They are given a fixed payment per patient to keep the patient as healthy as possible. Several of these plans have demonstrated that focusing on *patient outcomes* rather than *billable services* can be a win-win-win situation: the patients stay healthier, the physicians have a better work environment without a reduction in compensation, and the insurer (CMS in this case) saves money. As I mentioned, this model could apply to many system environments.

Conversion to such an outcomes-based rather than a service-based model is not easy. It will be fraught with mistakes requiring revision and will make many providers anxious. I tried to cast a vision for such a model in one large system. We had the infrastructure to accomplish it. However, the specialty providers were concerned that we were trying to turn them all into primary care providers. Of course, in such a model, procedures, testing, and specialty care will be largely unchanged (since the patients are unchanged). But instead of striving to do more procedures and check more CPT code boxes, we would be doing what was needed to optimize outcomes, not just for individual patients but for our whole service area. And we could afford to spend more time on community-building activities!

Be Attentive to the Greater Community

I would be remiss if I did not expand the sense of community to the actual communities in which healthcare systems work. The residents in our service area care about their healthcare options. I am fortunate to live in Cleveland, Ohio. The overall quality of care in our city is very high due in part to the Case Western Reserve Medical School and also the Cleveland Clinic Health System, University Hospitals Health System, and MetroHealth Medical Center. It would be hard to find anyone who has not heard of one of these institutions and the associated excellence in the healthcare they provide. The Cleveland Clinic has worked hard to be a part of the larger Cleveland community, and the community has rewarded that commitment with a sense of pride. Patients from all over love informing me that they get their care at the Cleveland Clinic.

I have also worked in hospital systems with a poor reputation in their surrounding community. How these reputations developed is varied but in each case reflects a failure of the system to prioritize the importance of their providers and the quality of care they deliver.

The breadth of care delivered is not the critical factor. (After all, not every hospital can or should offer every service.) Still, those services they offer should be done with excellence, and they should be actively engaged in assessing how the residents perceive the care they or their loved ones receive. In some of these communities, the residents actively avoid the local hospital.

Steps You Can Take

Build time for group interaction, interdisciplinary rounds, town hall meetings, social gatherings, weekly section meetings, etc.
Any of these will go a long way to building community in your organization. This will require a top-down cultural shift; it must be made clear that these activities are encouraged and important.

Apply tools to gauge the sense of community in your system.
The SCI is a good start.[20] Another is Linzer's OWL survey.[21] Use the results to design improvements and then remeasure.

Encourage your organization to use the Gallup Q12 assessment tool.[22]
If you can't get approval for a system-wide survey, start with one in your own department or office setting.

Include input from varied members of the organization on as many decision points as possible.
This will build a sense of influence and buy-in.

Align administration and provider goals (and, if possible, compensation).
Limit these to a few each year so that multiple inclusive community-building activities can be created around them.

Listen to each other.
Every person should have a voice and be respected.

Be transparent.

Share data and metrics in an open and timely fashion. Likewise, when system problems are investigated, communicate the corrective action plan and get buy-in.

Consider if you could implement some outcome-based metrics into your system.

Offset the concern of compensation loss by rewarding better outcomes.

Things to Avoid:

Don't ignore the emotional and social aspects of the workforce in the name of efficiency.

Every administrator will agree that the cost of recruiting and training a new provider is enormous. Far better and less costly to build in some community-building time, forgoing some billing activities.

Don't focus only on activities that generate current income.

Rather, foster creative thinking about how the organization could evolve and do better. Include the providers in working on solving system issues.

Don't develop administrative (or worse yet, consultant company) solutions that are then forced upon the providers.

This is the fastest way to set up an "us vs. them" mentality!

Don't forget that the sense of community shared by your organization greatly influences the perception of your organization by your surrounding patient population.

It is much easier to create a good impression than to repair an unfavorable one.

Specific Implementation Tips:

Academic Centers

- *Reinvigorate the daily educational activities with morning conferences attended by all.* Make this an expectation, and design ways for both seasoned and junior staff to contribute.
- *Sponsor bimonthly provider social events.* For example, our department has a regular story-slam with poetry readings, short skits, or other creative exhibits around a potluck meal.
- *Encourage and provide protected time for section meetings.*
- *Hold a once-yearly retreat where every provider participates.* This may require using outside resources to cover essential services for a day. Plan the event carefully to address felt needs expressed by the providers. Then, follow up with regular committee meetings to address action items.
- *If your system has multiple hospitals, design and install a mechanism for all providers to participate in person or remotely for the same meeting.* Current networking solutions make this easy to accomplish. Rotate the host location so all sites are included.
- *Provide monthly evaluations for providers focused on*

  - setting or reevaluating expectations;
  - encouraging or rewarding or celebrating successes;
  - addressing and exploring solutions for felt staffing or equipment needs; and
  - providing unique support for provider-stated goals (e.g., training course, coaching, mentorship). Actively empower and support personal growth.

Community Hospitals

- *Actively encourage and provide support for medical staff meetings and functions.*
- *Actively encourage social events involving both providers and administrators.* With the exception of my dyad colleagues, I can

never recall being invited to lunch by an administrator at one of my hospitals.

- *Set up hospital-wide group activities and encourage provider participation.* I still remember seeing the CEO and the chief of staff of a community hospital with aprons on serving ice cream to the nurses and staff!

- *Establish regular meetings to update providers on hospital metrics and performance.* Use these opportunities to garner input and opinions from providers. While there is often an administrative report given at staff meetings, I have rarely seen any effort to have open discussion or interaction. Unlike business professionals, providers may need some encouragement to participate.

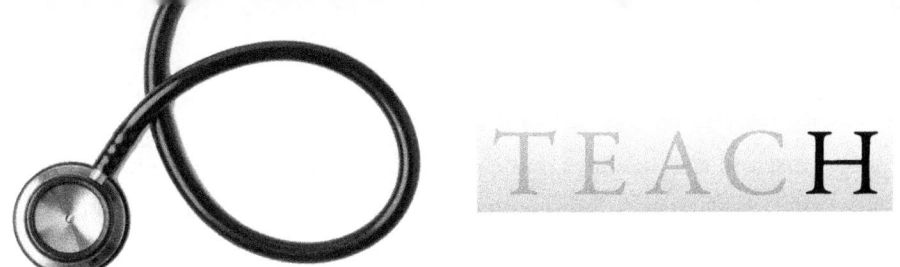

TEAC**H**

Chapter 8

Practicing Honor

Honor is an interesting concept. Different people define it differently. For some, it could mean a special event to celebrate an accomplishment. It could be an attitude of being open to another's opinion or perspective. Or maybe it conjures an approach to those perceived as possessing more wisdom, power, or experience. I like to think of honor as our response to a God-given innate worth in other persons. People deserve to be honored because they are all worthy of that attitude. Thus, I can honor my experienced mentor but just as easily honor my chronically ill disabled patient. And as providers, we like to be honored as well! When we do not feel valued at work or feel we are treated unfairly, that is being dishonored.

Removal of Clerical Assistance

Providers have been dishonored in one way that has been very subtle and insidious. We used to have clerical assistance. When I first started in practice, I had an assistant assigned to me as their only provider. They handled correspondence, phone calls, manuscript preparation, and database updates. Marilyn is still a good friend, and I still see her from time to time at the hospital. Over time, these positions have been gradually eliminated. Most recently, I was assigned to an assistant who also had eight other providers to attend to. Technology has enabled some of this shift. Central scheduling services, which have their own issues, word processing software, dictation voice recognition programs, and the like have made many tedious processes easier. Thus, tasks that our assistant used to handle have now been reassigned to us. No longer do I have someone filtering my in-box; I have to do that online in the EMR. No longer does someone prepare my manuscripts or budget spreadsheets; I am expected to do this myself on my computer. I no longer have someone I can turn to and ask to connect me with a referring doctor; I have to search for them on Google myself. Instead of doing what I do best—and what only I can do (provide patient care)—I am now expected to perform tasks I was not trained to do or are not the best use of my time.

On the one hand, I long for the community and teaming I had with prior assistants, but being a very tech-savvy person, I am quite capable of managing these extra assignments. However, many of my colleagues struggle with keeping their in-boxes cleared and their charts closed. At one point, I had to build financial incentives or holdbacks into the compensation package to encourage these activities. If these tasks could be assigned to a nursing partner or an advanced practitioner, it might be a better use of everyone's time. While I believe many of these software-based changes are positive and here to stay, I feel we need to acknowledge that many providers feel dishonored by being expected to do clerical tasks.

EMR Inhibition of Communication

Dishonoring often occurs in many small ways. Each event is easily excusable by itself, but it can be frustrating when they frequently occur throughout the day. Here are a few examples from a single day.

My first patient for catheterization was hospitalized overnight and on heparin. I specifically noted in the orders and mentioned to their nurse when I left that evening that I wanted the heparin to continue without interruption. On arrival at the catheterization laboratory, it is evident that their heparin was stopped three hours prior!

I previously gave the laboratory staff a detailed description (written) of how I like my back table set up and what equipment I typically use. When I got to the table, none of that information had been incorporated.

Later, I wrote an order for a beta-blocker and specifically noted in the comments that I did not want it to be held for any particular low heart rate. The patient's heart rate runs in the mid-50s, and the nurse held her beta-blocker.

I also ordered a long-acting preparation to be given twice daily and noted that I did in fact want it twice daily in the comments section of the order. Twenty minutes later, I was called by the pharmacist to inform me that I ordered a long-acting preparation twice daily instead of once. They didn't bother to read the comments.

I specifically ordered a follow-up appointment to be made in two weeks with the referring provider, not me. At the time of discharge, I noted that the appointment was made with *me* for the next week. The ward clerk assumed I would want to see them personally. They didn't bother to read the order either.

These events occur despite written specifics to the contrary. They reflect a lack of attention to detail and reflect the lost impact of teaming and community. If I'm expected to use the EMR for everything (verbal orders are now frowned upon or banned altogether), then my use of it needs to be honored! I am not against others checking my orders to ensure accuracy or to look out for possible drug interactions, but the events I described are all acts of failure to honor specific written directions.

Honoring with Honest Feedback

I remember a radiology technician working in our laboratory many years ago. When I met to give her a yearly evaluation, she was shocked that my ratings were not as high as those she had received in the past. A long discussion and a few tears ensued, but it was worth it. I explained and gave concrete examples of some behaviors that could be improved. She was able to recognize these behaviors and understand how she could improve. She had not received honest feedback during her prior evaluations. While you might think she would become bitter after this encounter, she actually was thankful for the feedback and worked to improve. She became one of my strongest advocates and best workers!

When delivered in a safe environment and in a nonthreatening way, most colleagues would rather have an honest evaluation than one with little thought. Feedback can be positive as well. I recently noticed a hospitalist colleague who wrote excellent notes in the EMR. I sought him out to compliment and tell him that I appreciated the extra effort he was expending to make his notes informative and thoughtful. It caught him off guard, but after his initial surprise, he was very thankful. Most of our EMR feedback comes from the hospital coders and billers, and it is rarely complimentary! I encourage you to make an effort to spend the few minutes required to compliment a job well done. All of us can use the lift it creates in our busy day.

Honoring Our Colleagues' Career Goals

Many years ago, I recognized the potential of a young ward clerk on the telemetry unit. I encouraged her often and suggested she work on a nursing degree. When I moved to another city, she was still a ward clerk; however, when I returned twelve years later, she was a registered nurse working in the unit. After a few more years, I supported her application for the head nurse of the coronary care unit. She is doing an outstanding job and encouraging the next generation of leaders.

At a small community hospital where I worked, a radiology technician who had grown up and started her family in town was always supportive of the new program we were starting. I tried to give her special projects, and she always completed them with excellence. Eventually, the service line director position became vacant, and she was considering applying. I counseled her on the politics of such a position and really pressed her on whether she wanted those headaches with a growing family. She assured me she could handle it, and she was correct! She is doing a great job as the cardiovascular service line director, and her can-do attitude and local knowledge are boosting her career.

A medical resident from Pakistan training in a nearby community hospital program spent a week at our academic center on the consult service. By chance, I was the attending for that week (the only week I did all year). He outshone all of the theoretically better-trained university residents and fellows in both his fund of knowledge and his diligence in studying to understand each medical condition. He would bring in research articles every morning and teach us about the patient conditions we encountered. During the same week, I was asked to write a review article about using a specialized cardiology device. I was so impressed with him that I offered for him to write it with me. He came to my office and took home a few review articles I had in my files to see if it was of interest. He arrived the next day and was eager to get started. We developed an outline for the manuscript, and then the week was over. To my surprise, a week later, I received a typed thirty-page manuscript with 180 full references. It needed a little work prior to submission, but he had demonstrated his commitment. We published the manuscript, and then I was able to help him secure fellowships so he could follow his dream to be an interventional cardiologist. I honored his work ethic and intelligence, not his past training or stature.

When I was on sabbatical in Germany, a young *Arzt im Praktikum* (AiP), the equivalent of a US intern, worked in cardiology. He was brilliant and very adept at research. He did the majority of the work for a research project, and I gave him first author status on our resulting manuscript. Making an AiP first author is unheard of in Germany, but I insisted on honoring his effort over the objections of the hospital director (who, by the way, authored the definitive German cardiology textbook). That AiP, Dr. Mueller, is now an accomplished professor of medicine in Basel, Switzerland, and a lifelong friend. He has published several times in the most prestigious journals in our field.

These experiences have been especially rewarding for me. However, the support I gave was not the result of original concepts formed by me. I fully remember the eighth-grade math teacher who encouraged me, the professor of physiology in medical school who supported my early cardiovascular research, and my first cardiac ICU attending who encouraged my passion for the heart. Never underestimate the importance of encouragement and honor from a senior mentor!

Honoring by Inviting Colleagues to Share in Our Lives

Another way to honor our colleagues is to invite them into your life.

My wife and I have often taken in hors d'oeuvres and sparkling grape juice on New Year's Eve to celebrate with the night shift nurses and residents. While they might have had a tray of goodies delivered by the hospital nutrition staff, it did not have nearly the impact of the director and his wife coming in at 11:30 p.m. to celebrate with them personally!

We have tried to have two yearly events at our home for the fellows, lab staff, and their guests. We would host a barbecue event in the summer with games, beer, and burgers. To make it special, we would bring in an ice cream truck or entertainment for the kids. In the winter, we would host a formal gala at our home with a nice catered dinner and holiday games. We would have something special planned for the adults as well: a harpist or a string quartet, for example. It was fun for everyone to get dressed up—quite a change from masks and caps. Often, I could hardly recognize some of the staff! We would talk and play interactive games or respond to interesting questions. One especially fun activity was watching them decorate a colleague as a Christmas tree person. They gathered lights, ornaments, garland, and tinsel and adorned one of their colleagues. To see several teams competing for the best "tree" was hilarious!

Caring for Our Environment Honors Everyone

I believe a pleasing environment leads to better attitudes. I have purchased nature photos to place in front of the stress treadmill machines. It gives our patients something to look at while they are running and a focal point to discuss with the nurse supervising the test. It took very little effort to find matching artwork for our office walls and silk floral arrangements to brighten our counters. Unless you practice in a very upscale institution, you know that decorating is a low priority. Nothing prevents providers from helping in this regard. It costs little but makes the environment more professional and conveys the idea that we care about our surroundings. If a patient sees that we keep our own space in order, how much more reassured will they be that we will also keep their health in order.

Much to the dismay of the hospital's facility department, I once repainted some accent walls in our intensive care unit. I came in one evening with drop cloths, rollers, and tape, and in about two hours, the scuffed and discolored walls were revitalized. I also took home and repaired the pictures that had fallen off the wall. Yes, I got in trouble! But I was tired of the impression our disheveled unit appearance gave to the patients and their visitors. In fact, I had two patients and their families who refused to stay at our hospital for needed bypass surgery given the unkempt surroundings on the unit. After two years of unanswered work orders, I decided to use my other talents to brighten things up. In some ways this was rebellious, but in others it was an act of frustration at being ignored for several years. I wanted to be part of the solution! No one disagreed that the place needed a freshening up, and I had the skills to do it, so why not help? I guess unions and liability are the why not. I just wanted to honor the staff and patients with a pleasant work environment that reflected the excellent medical care we delivered.

Honoring Our Colleagues' Involvement in Key Administrative Issues
As I discussed in a previous chapter, involvement in administration is important. I think this is also a way to honor our colleagues. When I was a department chair, I established a council made up of provider leaders from each of the departments' sections, six persons total. We would meet for two hours monthly, and I ensured that this time was protected from all other duties. The purpose was to give them insight into department issues, solicit suggestions for solutions, and empower them to function as local sources of information for their sections. I thought this would be an honor for them. I was wrong.

Many seemed frustrated that I was making them do yet another task. They were frustrated that I asked them to study issues and provide feedback and suggestions. They were frustrated that they had to drive an hour to meet on some occasions. I see this as a cultural failure. They had never been afforded this degree of insight and responsibility and were only expected to get their clinical work done. I learned that it was hard to honor them with administration without the foundation of teamwork, equity, and community.

Institutional Events That Show Honor

I have also experienced refreshing examples of institutional-honoring events.

One hospital that had been present in the community for over 150 years had a Hall of Fame. Physician leaders were honored by being included in this public display with a portrait and a plaque describing their contributions to medicine, the hospital, and the community. New members were inducted into the Hall of Fame with a formal ceremony. At this same facility, a senior physician and prior department chair had spent his entire career dedicated to research and teaching generations of young physicians and nurses. We honored him by rededicating and renaming the cardiac ICU after him.

Recently, I was honored at this same hospital. I had been working there when I received my professorship from the Case Western Reserve University. We were honored at a nice gathering with an embroidered stole indicating our academic achievement. With it came a handwritten note from the chief of medicine, who was a longtime friend of mine. To my knowledge, this was the first event of its kind at the institution. It was a very thoughtful reminder of an achievement that had occurred sixteen years earlier.

At a different large teaching hospital, a young colleague of mine worked tirelessly to secure a position among the first to implant percutaneous aortic valves. She organized the complex team necessary to pull this off and established a robust referral and vetting process for prospective patients. After the first successful patient implant, she honored the entire team by arranging a professional photo shoot and write-up in the local papers complimenting the entire team's effort!

Institutional-honoring events don't have to be this formal, however. At a small community hospital, there was a monthly gathering with cake or cookies to honor all of the staff with birthdays that month. Simple and cheap, but a very effective way to indicate that someone cared about you as a person.

I have also been privileged to be involved in over twenty-five years of a prominent interventional cardiology conference. While the live case demonstrations, lectures, and research presentations have always been exciting, I found the institution of the Lifetime Achievement Award to be the most gratifying part of the program. Each year, one of the world leaders in the field was honored in a prolonged ceremony involving a montage video, colleague testimonials, and family celebration. It was wonderful to see the packed room each year as one of our colleagues was honored.

> Going out of your way to help others feel valued and respected will go a long way toward healing a broken system.

In this chapter, I've outlined some specific, intentional ways we can honor each other with many examples of how I've tried to honor people throughout my career. Yes, it takes effort to honor people, but the results are worth it. Some of the simplest ways I try to honor people are often the most well received, like honoring my patients by being on time for my appointments and giving them my phone number to use for emergencies. They have never abused that honor, and in fact, the very few calls I have received have usually been to share their appreciation! I show honor to the nursing staff by bringing in fresh flowers for no specific reason. I try not to do doughnuts, since we all claim to be on diets. I honor the nurses who work with me by seeking them out personally to inform them of changes or important objectives for my patients. If a referring physician sends me a new patient, I honor them by sending a handwritten thank-you note. I honor my coworkers by encouraging their career advancement, being on time for appointments, and providing honest and timely feedback. I show honor to my colleagues in the medical industry by being on time for appointments and being honest in my feedback to them as well. Remember, everyone deserves honor. Going out of your way to help others feel valued and respected will go a long way toward healing a broken system.

Steps You Can Take

Establish teams that can share the administrative or clerical burden with the providers.
Often a dedicated medical assistant and an advanced practitioner can deal with the bulk of routine communication.

Acknowledge the need for occasional breaks from clinical activity.
Build these breaks into the provider schedules.

Be responsive to provider requests.
We are intelligent adults and can understand the conflicting requirements of any system. We do not appreciate being ignored, however. If the system cannot respond to a request, just be honest and say so. And don't be afraid to solicit input from the provider to explore potential solutions to specific requests.

Establish recurring events that honor the provider staff.
These events do not have to be elaborate, but with the many metrics we now collect, there are multiple ways to honor those who provide exceptional care or go above and beyond for their patients. Make sure these events are public and inclusive.

On a system level, work with other leaders to explore more honoring traditions, like the Hall of Fame or Lifetime Achievement Awards I described above.
I often see portraits of prior hospital board members or large donors, but rarely anything to do with providers!

Things to Avoid:

Don't fill every moment of the day with clinical activities.
Providing some scheduled free time allows for providers to catch up with charting or accommodate unexpectedly ill or complex patients without feeling stressed.

Don't exclude providers from those worthy of special honor in hospital systems.
While the board members, administrators, and donors are important, physician leaders are equally deserving of honor and recognition.

Specific Implementation Tips

Academic Centers

- *Block thirty minutes in midmorning and midafternoon and forty-five to sixty minutes at noon in provider schedules to allow for some decompression time.*
- *If evening or weekend schedules are appropriate for patient access, don't expect the provider to work a full weekday schedule.*
- *Establish leadership councils to provide an outlet for provider education and input regarding the clinical operation.*
- *Establish a Hall of Fame for providers who have contributed greatly to the organization.* This could be for the entire institution, but consider implementing this in each department as well to spread the effect.
- *Look for young, promising colleagues.* Encourage and promote them in their career path.
- *Advocate for the support staff.* Go to bat to get them a nice work environment, good equipment, and decent compensation. They are employed to care for our patients and provide the testing we request. Show your appreciation by acknowledging what's important for them.

Community Hospitals

- *Establish several monthly events that honor providers.* This could include the birthday idea or recognition of high performance on patient satisfaction scores, timely chart completion, or a patient success story.
- *As above, advocate for the support staff!*
- *Establish community-included events that honor providers.* This could take the form of educational gatherings at local clubs or facilities where providers describe and answer questions about their specialty. Among the many hospitals I have worked at, only one had an active community liaison. She was constantly setting me up for talks and visits with both referring providers and community groups. It made me feel that my presence was important to the hospital.
- *Establish one or two events each year that are specifically designed to honor providers and their families.* One small hospital hosted a party in a senior provider's home to introduce and acclimate new providers every August.

Part Three

Becoming Effective Leaders

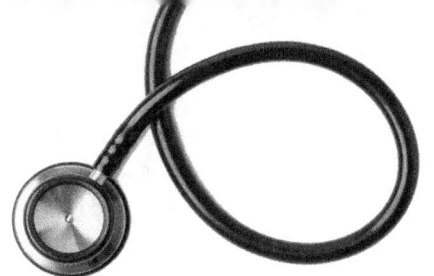

Chapter 9

The Provider's Responsibility

So far, I have described ways the healthcare system has impacted providers and have given some simple and inexpensive changes that could restore provider fulfillment and excitement. While the system, along with regulations and payment schemes, has undoubtedly made our lives less enjoyable, we are not exempt from blame for the current situation. In my experience, providers have abdicated their responsibility in many situations. We are, after all, central to healthcare delivery and not helpless or powerless to promote change! In some cases, we have abused the system to our advantage; in others, we have become egocentric and entitled.

To be respected as part of a solution to the dysfunction in healthcare, we must set the example and take responsibility. Four key character traits are fundamental to providers being empowered to improve the system: humility, accountability, integrity, and leadership. I believe it is important to discuss these and to own our part in the current dysfunction. Before I get into these topics, and to help you understand the basis for my perspective, let me share my story with you.

My Story

Where I was born doesn't exist anymore. In 1953, my father, Jack, was deployed with Naval Intelligence in Alaska. I'm not sure he was in one of those if-I-told-you-I'd-have-to-kill-you jobs, but it was enough to keep him on station when I was born at the North Island Naval

Hospital in Coronado, California. Thankfully, although the hospital has long since been demolished, the famed Hotel Coronado still reminds me of those earliest days of learning to walk in the breezy sun of Southern California! We moved often during my childhood due to my father striving for higher education in New York City, student teaching, and then securing his big opportunity as a school principal in upstate New York. My brother (three years junior) was born, and we were by all accounts a typical postwar family of the 1950s.

Then, in the summer of 1960, my path into medicine was abruptly placed before me. My father died quite quickly from Hodgkin's Lymphoma at the age of thirty. As a seven-year-old, I became the man of the house. I distinctly remember the surgeon general's warning in 1963 that smoking caused cancer. That was when I determined (unconsciously at first) to stamp out disease.

With both parents being educators and having a librarian for a grandmother, I found it easy to devote myself to my studies, and I was fortunate to ultimately finish medical school in 1978. This was during the dawn of the subspecialty we now call interventional cardiology. I was drawn to the combination of technical/surgical skills and medicine/physiology needed to perform balloon angioplasty and care for acute myocardial infarction patients.

I was also drawn to a beautiful, life-filled young nursing student named Dinah. She was a senior in the three-year, hospital-based program run by the hospital where I was training. We met in a psychology therapy group for nursing and medical students and have shared the rest of our story together. She largely raised our three wonderful children and has supported me in my career climb—the many moves (about fifteen), the frequent travel, and the late nights on call. She has since become an ordained pastor, counselor, and writer. And now she is

> To be respected as part of a solution to the dysfunction in healthcare, we must set the example and take responsibility.

finishing her PhD! She has been critical to me, my career, our children, and our shared adventures.

My career has not been static—anything but! I have been driven by the deep-seated notion instilled as a seven-year-old to make a difference in the health of my patients (after all, I couldn't with my father). Being driven can be good, but it can also be overwhelming at times. Learning to balance the drive with compassion, listening skills, and relationships has been a lifelong exercise, one I have failed at frequently. At each stage in my career, I have tried to extract the best lessons and build forward on them. I have also pursued my goals in four seemingly unrelated spheres of life: interventional cardiology, professional education, health-related missions, and entrepreneurship. Each sphere has taught me important lessons, and each has informed my thinking and opinions on the topics in this book. They are so intertwined that trying to separate them is futile and frankly serves no purpose.

Let me touch on a few highlights of the journey. After fellowship, my first official job was in the VA healthcare system. I had an encouraging mentor who fostered my desire to study physiology and provided the time and tools to allow me to set up an experimental lab. During those four years, I also began working with industry partners to develop tools needed for the new field of interventional cardiology. I was fortunate to be among the first to develop and use intravascular ultrasound in patients, allowing detailed views of the inside of blood vessels. This ultimately led to many publications, worldwide travel, and presentations. At his request, I followed my mentor to my next academic job in Cleveland, Ohio. There I developed training programs, continued my experimental and human investigation, and supervised a team of nurses, technicians, and trainees. I assisted in the design of a new hospital and helped develop a robust clinical trials operation. Our family spent a year on sabbatical in the Black Forest of Germany. In Germany, I experienced a very different style of medicine, one that was more relaxed but also incredibly efficient, more focused on relationships, yet quite productive. It was there that I learned that clinical excellence and authentic relationships *could* coexist!

After returning to Cleveland, I assisted a colleague in building a large cardiology program at a tertiary care county hospital. I was subsequently offered the chance to start a heart and vascular institute at a large community hospital in another city. Unfortunately, I learned that the academic-employed model I enjoyed was not appreciated by all my peers. Our effort to develop the institute was sincere but ultimately unsuccessful. Wanting to allow my daughter to finish high school in that city, I started a concierge cardiology practice. The recession of 2008 was not an opportune time to do so! As you might imagine, with incomes falling and house foreclosures the norm, patients were not eager to sign up. So we toughed it out for two years, then returned to the East Coast academic environment. I was offered the cardiology chairmanship at a large integrated health system. While not university affiliated, it was academically oriented. I learned about the incredible advantages that can be realized by influencing all three parts of the healthcare system: provider practice, hospital services, and insurance.

Ultimately, Dinah and I moved back to the Cleveland area to be near our children. I was able to work in the same academic center I had left fifteen years prior. I have also been able to work for an organization that provides cardiology services for smaller hospitals that cannot support hiring multiple physicians to provide interventional services. From foreign to domestic, rural to urban, not-for-profit to for-profit, community to academic, and small to large, I have experienced the gamut of health systems. I have tried to be a good student and learn ways to improve the system from each experience.

When not at work, we participated in medical mission trips as a family. My wife and I felt it important to expose our kids to the "real world" outside the United States. In the early 1990s, my daughter (who was eighteen months old) slept in a suitcase and a backpack while my wife ran triage in a small mountain town in Honduras. My five-year-old son entertained the local children and escorted patients from triage to the exam area. My eight-year-old son helped in the "pharmacy" packaging meds into baggies for the patients. I worked with an interpreter and a dentist to deliver whatever care we could manage. Trips to Haiti,

Nigeria, Ghana, Benin, South Africa, Swaziland, Thailand, Peru, and Russia followed over the years. By the time they graduated from high school, my children had been in over thirty countries. Most importantly, these trips kept us humbly aware of the incredible healthcare opportunities we have in the United States.

My educational efforts grew into several small companies developing educational software for healthcare professionals. With an engineering colleague, we developed image interpretation software. With another very talented programmer, we wrote award-winning interactive training programs using the internet in the days before smartphones and apps. Our mission work grew into board positions with several organizations and multimillion-dollar Centers for Disease Control and Prevention grants to promote childhood health in sub-Saharan Africa and India. My clinical and academic experiences led to wonderful friendships with medical leaders around the world and influential positions on writing groups and with professional societies. My time training cardiologists worldwide in interventional techniques again exposed me to a wide range of healthcare systems in foreign countries spanning Europe, the Middle East, India, South America, and Asia.

I have one younger (and smarter) brother who has been involved in private equity investing since 1982. Fifteen years ago, I convinced my brother that we should be investing in start-up companies in the healthcare space. I looked for interesting ideas, and he provided the business acumen. We have had some minor successes but many more failures! I have seen what works, what does not, and how hard it is to get even great ideas through the maze of regulatory and marketing hurdles to successful commercialization. I also have learned that regardless of how novel or exciting the technology may be, creating a successful company depends far more on the leadership guiding the effort. Leadership skills are key, not only in business but in healthcare. That important topic will be our focus in chapter 13.

I mention these varied experiences not as a measure of accomplishment. In truth, some of these efforts and experiences did not end as hoped, and some failed miserably. I offer them as evidence of a persistent desire to understand how we can provide an environment that combines clinical excellence, business acumen, and compassion. One that any of us would be proud to be affiliated with, care for our patients in, and not be concerned to recommend for our own families. I hope that my experiences garnered from varied institutions, spheres of life, and the global community can shed light on the current healthcare situation and empower each of us to make a difference. If you are reading this as a healthcare provider, many of you have similar stories. All of you are dedicated and hard working. We all have high-functioning capacity, so I know we can create a better environment. We can recapture the missional culture of healthcare delivery. It is our responsibility to do so!

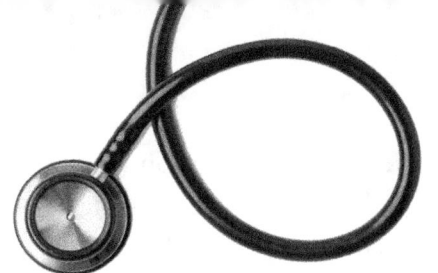

Chapter 10

Humility

H umility is a tough one for providers. We are used to excelling in school and in life by all external standards. We have typically been the "smart kids"—the ones who did well on standardized tests, were asked to be in advanced placement classes, and now get to wear the shining white coats that shout "doctor in the house!"

I once worked with a physician leader. He had many forward-thinking ideas and achieved success for the institution, but he did so without a bit of humility. He was often very condescending and engaged in profanity-laced reprimands. Those who worked for him were not enabled but controlled. Ultimately, many very capable and more personable leaders left the institution. His lack of humility overshadowed the many positive accomplishments of the institution. In the universe of providers, he is unfortunately not alone. Many providers have excelled due to their strengths and intelligence but missed greater opportunities due to their lack of humility.

Humility, however, does not mean downplaying our strengths but, rather, being honest about our abilities. I talked about LeBron James earlier. If he were to say, *I'm not very good at basketball*, we would immediately recognize that this is false humility. Similarly, if a surgeon is excellent at a particular procedure, it is OK for that skill to be recognized. What matters is how you handle that reality. In professional football, there is now a taunting penalty for those players who like to rub their achievements into the opponents' faces. Similarly, providers do not need to be arrogant or aloof about their personal abilities. Humility is recognizing the special talents or abilities you have, being honest about them, but not unnecessarily promoting them.

Staff Interactions

One important lesson I have learned is that providers need to be especially careful about how they interact with hospital staff. We fail to recognize that being a provider places us in a position of authority that colors our interactions with everyone else in the healthcare system. A statement we make in jest with another provider can easily be interpreted negatively when made to a nursing colleague or a patient aide. Even when we do not want to be viewed this way, it comes with the title, and we need to be aware of it in every interaction. In my experience, it takes several months of working together with my nursing colleagues to be comfortable engaging in small talk. Before they get to know me, there is always a bit of hesitancy that I might be looking to criticize them or get them in trouble. If you have a more direct personality, as I do, seemingly innocent questions about patient status can be misinterpreted as accusatory. I have had to learn to preface my questions with the statement that I am confused and just looking for clarification.

Another potential for misunderstanding arises during emergencies. During a code blue, rapid response, or procedure emergency, the provider must assume responsibility and direct the ensuing sequence of events. We are legally and morally responsible for the welfare of our patients. We need to be decisive, direct, and clear in our management of the situation. Our direct approach can sometimes be misinterpreted as insensitive, unprofessional, or demeaning. Several situations can help lessen this effect. First, having a preexisting relationship with the other emergency participants provides relationship capital that offsets the acute, uncomfortable situation. Second, a post-event debrief session can go a long way to explaining your concern for the process, your reasons for the actions taken, and the feelings of the other participants. Humility can be demonstrated by acknowledging that the situation was unsettling and that your actions were directed toward helping the patient and were never intended to make the staff feel uncomfortable. In my experience, these debrief situations can enhance trust and break down false impressions. Our colleagues all want what is best for the patient and are relieved to understand that our goal as providers is in absolute alignment. A provider who is unprepared or unsure during emergencies is likely to be viewed even more harshly by the staff. Our responsibility is to be prepared and, if we are unsure, seek rapid counsel from others, not just try to bluster our way through. Saying honestly, "I don't know what to do" and asking for help demonstrates humility.

Too many providers spend more time complaining about patient care than they do trying to improve the care. Our role as providers is to teach, encourage, and be part of a team. If a patient call light is on, providers can attend to that. If a nurse is unclear about a postoperative issue, providers can sit and explain it to them. Suppose a family member arrives late and needs clarification of their loved one's condition. In that case, providers can take the time to address their concerns, even if you just finished talking to the other family members! Nothing should be beneath us. Humility is being willing to give our time and expertise to those who are less comfortable with the complexities of what we do. Yes, hands-on nursing care has declined in the era of EHR and endless documentation, but we can still instruct, encourage, and assist. We can set the example and help our colleagues develop into more effective caregivers.

In earlier chapters, I talked about key features of a healthy system. Being part of a team, having equity in the system, and having a good sense of community make it easier for us to practice humility. Sometimes, as often happens with me, our initial interactions upon starting in a new work environment may be misinterpreted. However, the chance of misinterpretation decreases rapidly once we are part of the team and have integrated into the community. Learning the "rules" of the environment takes some time and often comes with some missteps. One mechanism to accelerate your assimilation is to find an understanding teammate. This could be another provider or one of the staff you will regularly interact with. Having at least one person willing to support you as you get used to the environment will reduce your anxiety level significantly. Over time you will become more invested in the system. When this happens, you will naturally work harder to fit into the culture and participate as part of the team.

Being Humble with Patients

A potentially difficult dynamic exists for provider interactions with patients and their families. Providers are viewed as powerful, influential, and nearly unquestionable. We need to take every opportunity to diffuse this power imbalance. Several simple steps can help. Whenever possible, sit down when addressing patients. If need be, roll in a chair from the nursing station. You can sit on the bed in a pinch, but never without asking the patient's permission first. Their bed is the only piece of the system they have any control over! Introduce yourself and give the patient a business card or write your name down. Speak slowly and look in their eyes when you talk. Use terms and analogies that they can understand. This may vary depending on the patient's education or profession, but never assume that anyone understands the specific jargon that is common among providers. When a provider is my patient, I am even more careful not to assume anything! Always ask the patient (and their family) if they understand what you are saying, and never leave without asking if they have any further questions or needs. You may be busy, but when you visit a patient, they must feel like they have your full attention. And be transparent; if you need to attend to another urgent issue, just say so. They will understand.

Most importantly, never lie to a patient or their family. If the news is bad, you can soften it, but it must be said. If a complication has occurred, be the first to mention it. If you misjudged something, admit your failing. While the risk managers may not want us admitting fault, it is fine to admit that you are sorry when things do not go as planned. Thankfully, I have not had very many serious procedural complications, but I have certainly dealt with many dying patients and their grieving families in dealing with heart disease. Some of the worst cases are those resuscitated from sudden death but remaining in a coma. Walking with the family as they come to grips with the fact that their previously healthy loved one will not recover requires patience and a healthy dose of humility.

While we have statistics about chances of recovery, we cannot predict the future with certainty. Not long ago, a wife with a very strong level of faith was convinced that her husband would recover. He had collapsed in their backyard, and she watched in horror as the paramedics tried to resuscitate him. After some time, he did regain a rhythm but was in a deep coma. Despite initial attempts to preserve brain function, he was still comatose on day four. The odds were very poor, but we honored the wife's faith and supported the husband. About a week later, he woke up! He was subsequently transferred to a rehabilitation hospital and continued to improve. I had the honor to see him about a month later in the clinic. How humbling it was to walk with him into the ICU as he thanked the nurses who had cared for him despite all odds! Our commitment must remain to the patient and their family.

Faulty Perceptions

As providers, we need to be sensitive to perceptions and act rapidly to address them. If we sense that our actions have offended someone, we must stop and talk to them about it. It has become all too easy to use an online complaint form to describe interactions that we feel upset about. As professionals (and adults), we would be better served by a face-to-face interaction to address the issue and provide the opportunity for clarification and resolution. Doing so builds relationships and encourages humility. Anonymous online complaints are difficult to resolve and eliminate the opportunity for reconciliation. When things don't go as expected or a poor outcome occurs, face-to-face interaction is far more effective at understanding the technical and personal issues involved.

This has been a significant growth area for me. My focused, direct, logical approach can be interpreted as insensitive. Thus, I have adopted a strategy of reflecting on each interaction and making immediate amends if needed. I have made a point to gather the catheterization lab staff after stressful cases or those with complications. I make sure everyone has a chance to give their perceptions of what occurred and how they felt it was handled. I always ask for brutally honest feedback about my role in the situation. Did I make a mistake? Was I clear with my directions and orders? Did I overlook anything? I make a point to highlight how their actions were critical to our successes and also help them explore (in a nonjudgmental way) actions that have room for improvement. In my experience, these sessions allow us to relate as equals, where every opinion is valid. It also allows me to be seen in a different light. They recognize I make mistakes and have self-doubts just like they do. With that recognition comes a higher level of trust and community.

Honest Feedback

We all can benefit from feedback. During my early days working in the emergency room, I sent a self-addressed envelope with a paper questionnaire to the admitting physician for each patient I saw. I asked for some follow-up on the diagnosis and for suggestions on how I could improve my initial care. This was, of course, before EMR review or Survey Monkey allowed digital feedback. I have continued this willingness to get feedback by employing 360 reviews for my annual evaluations. Typically anonymous, they have provided wonderfully frank comments that become actionable for me. During every resident or fellow evaluation, I spend a healthy portion of our time getting their feedback on how I could be a better teacher and mentor for them. Unlike the practice in most corporate environments, receiving feedback on our personal interactions and areas for growth is unusual in the healthcare community. In my experience, systems providing regular provider-to-provider feedback are rare. You will probably have to seek this on your own. Otherwise, your feedback will typically only involve RVU production and queries about perceived poor care.

Receiving regular, honest feedback will keep you grounded and offer opportunities for self-improvement—more about this in chapter 13.

Broadening Your Horizons

Providers can also keep their humility in line by experiencing other environments or cultures. My travels have helped me to appreciate how fortunate we are in the United States to have excellent care. What we take for granted here is either nonexistent or a luxury in other countries. Let me share a few true experiences.

Can you imagine being the wife of a patient receiving a heart catheterization in Bangalore, India, and having the cardiologist come out of the laboratory and tell you that your husband needs a second stent, but you'll need to pay for it right then in advance? How could you say no? How stressful to try to find cash in a matter of minutes!

Can you imagine being in Swaziland and having a young volunteer working for you involved in an auto accident with a serious head injury? Before he can be transferred to a neighboring hospital in South Africa for emergency surgery, they require over $25,000 cash. No small ministry has that kind of money just sitting around, let alone in a third-world country!

Can you imagine a sixteen-year-old girl begging you to take out her remaining three decaying teeth because they are so painful? I experienced this in the hills of Honduras. For the lack of a toothbrush and toothpaste, she will experience a life without a beautiful smile. And, paradoxically, my son was having his teeth straightened with orthodontics on the same trip!

Imagine a young couple I know on vacation in Thailand. The husband has repeated seizures, and a CT scan shows a large brain tumor. Trying to fly him out for definitive care in the United States was a huge challenge and took nearly two weeks.

Every time I get upset about something not going perfectly with my patient's care, I try to remember those experiences and get my humility back in line.

As providers, we have demonstrated our intelligence, our commitment to study hard, and our willingness to work hard. With that demonstration comes recognition in a profession that carries a high level of respect and a comfortable income. If we stop there, however, we will miss out on even greater achievements. We cannot fully develop as influential leaders in our profession without a conscious effort to practice humility. We may accomplish tasks, but we will not leave a true legacy.

> We cannot fully develop as influential leaders in our profession without a conscious effort to practice humility.

Rarely will someone be remembered for solving an unusual diagnostic dilemma or performing a difficult surgery, but the one who was a humble team player dedicated to the patients and the system will have their name etched forever in the institutional memory.

Humility is not thinking less of yourself, it's thinking of yourself less.
—Rick Warren[23]

Steps You Can Take

Recognize that being a provider will color your interactions with others. Be very attentive to how you talk to those you work with to avoid appearing demeaning or aloof.

Recognize that you have a powerful position with your patients. Practice diffusing the power differential so that they feel supported and understood. Sit down when you interact. Make eye contact. Use understandable terms for them. Never lie. Be the first to admit missteps.

Invite honest feedback regarding your interactions and care. This could include a 360 evaluation. There are several simple-to-use platforms that can assist in accomplishing this type of evaluation. Or you can perform debrief sessions with your colleagues after stressful or complicated events.

Look for ways to be part of the solution to care.
Nothing should be beneath you.

If you are from a developed country, take time to reflect on how fortunate you are to work in modern healthcare systems.
It will help you keep perspective.

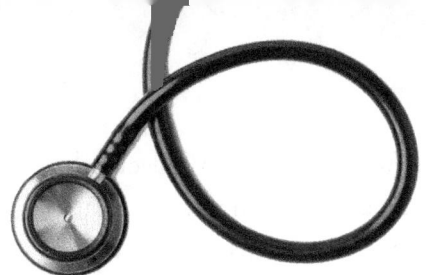

Chapter 11

Integrity

I once gave a lecture to young physicians in training. I used the analogy that integrity was like virginity—it's easy to lose but impossible to get back. As providers, we are expected to be highly professional, ethical, honest, and always have the patient's best interests at heart. We are expected to have integrity. When we act in ways that do not exemplify integrity, we degrade our entire profession. While I have failed in the humility arena on occasion, I have fortunately been able to maintain my integrity. One of my proudest moments was when a casual acquaintance introduced me to his colleagues at an industry meeting by saying that I demonstrated the highest level of integrity in our field. I certainly did not see that coming! It is something that I have always worked toward, and frankly, during times of fatigue or frustration, I came close to losing. So how can we as providers maintain our integrity? Let me share some experiences.

Integrity Must Be a Solemn Commitment

When I took the Hippocratic oath, I took it very seriously, just as I did my marriage vows. Only by this express commitment can we resist the temptations that will come our way. We will be seduced by money and power. It will start with small things but can escalate rapidly. Perhaps you own an imaging center as part of your practice. Since tests performed there can be reimbursed for both the technical and professional portions, there is a subtle temptation to order these tests to support your practice overhead. After all, if one can collect only $95 for an office visit but $1,000 for an ancillary test, you can appreciate the slippery slope of believing that these tests are all necessary. I don't think anyone sets out to be unethical, but when office bills are piling up and reimbursement is falling, more testing starts to seem reasonable as a way to make ends meet. We must resist that temptation. I have no problem with providers owning imaging centers. Non-guideline-directed self-referral, however, is a problem that gives our profession a bad name. Using one of many online tools to assess appropriateness is one way to prevent this. Another would be to submit to external accreditation or other review processes.

Taking director fees from institutions but not doing any work falls into the same category. Sounds like easy money, but it is wrong. I mentioned that a community hospital president once told me that they were paying over $12 million in "director" fees yearly. Wrong, wrong, wrong! These providers were not only taking director fees from that hospital but, in many cases, from two or three other facilities at the same time. In the vast majority of cases, a few JCAHO-mandated yearly meetings were held to justify the fees. The "directors" would show up for an hour to a meeting run by a hospital-employed nurse or administrator. The "directors" had no other substantive input that I could determine. Thankfully, the hospital realized this was a thinly veiled Stark Law violation and took steps to curtail the process! For those who are not aware, the Stark Law prohibits providers from referring patients to facilities if the provider has a financial relationship with the entity. The law was originally designed for healthcare systems that reimbursed providers on a fee-for-service basis. Providers rendering actual services at fair market value is not a violation, particularly when it is entirely unrelated to patient referral for services.

Lack of Integrity Does Not Have to Involve Money

Lack of integrity can be as simple as documenting in a note a physical exam you did not actually perform. The temptation to do this with the review of systems, exam, and history parts of our notes is immense.

These take time to do correctly, and our billing colleagues constantly flag these sections as inadequate. Many systems provide prepopulated forms. Despite this, such autopopulation actually constitutes Medicare fraud. We should never document services that we did not perform. Not only is it wrong, it undermines the main purpose of the note: to communicate accurate findings. We have all seen physical exam results documented on a ninety-year-old patient that would be hard to find in a normal sixteen-year-old athlete! In my opinion, it is far better to have a limited but accurate exam than a complete, largely fabricated one. The billing function of the note should be secondary; communication must remain primary.

Another example could be putting the nurses in a bad position by not agreeing to sign your verbal orders. Giving a verbal order is a de facto contract with the nurse. They agree to administer care, and you agree to document it later. Providers must honor their part of the contract. Another example could be making a mistake in ordering and blaming the nurse for the error. Many EMRs have multiple order choices, and despite what may appear to be accurate at first glance, the chosen order may not process properly. This gets back to my issue about proper orientation training and proper EMR maintenance. It's pretty frustrating when you think you ordered something, only to find out it never happened. This is not the nurse's fault. Despite the reason, the buck stops with the provider. Absent obvious misconduct by the nurse, responsibility for failure to communicate or failure to select the proper order falls on the provider. When these errors occur, assess the root cause and seek to educate or correct the issues. I find myself writing to the IT department several times a week to document flaws in the EMR system. Having integrity involves working to correct the issue, not just complaining about it.

A blatant example of a lack of integrity was when my colleagues in training would be on call for the training hospital but working during the same hours in a moonlighting job. Then, when they didn't answer the on-call pager, they would make up some excuse about how the pager was broken or the dog ate it! Another common issue occurs during handoff or shift change. How many times have you had to wait for the person relieving you? Being punctual is a sign of integrity. Some providers think they can get away with these things, especially justifying it by saying no one will be hurt or that their time is more valuable than others, but it is still wrong. We all know those few providers who have lost our trust due to repeated minor offenses indicating their lack of integrity.

Maintaining Integrity Requires Special Attention When We Are Fatigued

Without the underpinning of the solemn oath, we become especially vulnerable during times of fatigue. In my chosen subspecialty, I have been on call every three to four nights for patients arriving with a heart attack: the STEMI (ST-segment elevation myocardial infarction) call. After being up during the night in a stressful situation, it was not uncommon to have a full day of clinic visits or new patients to see in the hospital. The temptation to become superficial in my oversight of the inpatients, in my review of the new consult patient's chart, or in my attention to the clinic patient's stated issues was profound. Before each visit, I reminded myself that my fatigue did not justify the patient getting less of my focus and attention. It was a conscious and repetitive reminder as I worked through the day. Only after I was finished did I allow myself to get some rest. This may seem overly dramatic and a good example of the dysfunctional healthcare system demands. It is!

But as providers, we have an obligation to rise above the fatigue and give our patients our best effort. We are placed in a position of incredible influence and trust, so we must perform in a way deserving of the same. It is not the patient's fault that the system has not created an allowance for us to rest after being up all night. So until we find a way to solve that issue, we are bound by professional obligation to give each patient our best effort. If you experience these types of unrealistic work expectations, get involved and work with your colleagues to find a better solution! You are not helpless. Demonstrate integrity and work within the system to suggest positive solutions.

Integrity Must Be Maintained Outside of Our Patient Care Relationship

As professionals, we are often well known in our communities. How we interact with the grocery store clerk or the driver who cuts us off on our way into the parking lot also speaks to our integrity. This is intertwined with honor and humility. We providers put our pants on the same way as everyone else. We should get no special treatment. The truth is that others look up to us. They enjoy seeing us at the drycleaners and saying, "Hi, Doc!" They like introducing us to their family when we bump into them at the department store. How we act toward them and their friends in the community will impact our success. We should demonstrate the same integrity outside as we do inside the hospital. If someone forgets to include an item on our restaurant bill, we point it out and insist on paying the full amount. We don't buy items, use them, and then return them. We don't demand special rates or discounts, especially from those whom we know are far less financially sound than we are.

At one point, I was doing consulting for a manufacturer of X-ray equipment. They gave me a small grant to perform a study. For various reasons, we were never able to complete the study. I felt it only right to return the money, which I did. They were very thankful, even though it created a bit of an accounting problem for them. Return of grant money was a very infrequent occurrence! That simple act of integrity led to twenty more years of a great working relationship. Some years later, the same company instituted a program to have their sales force shadow us at work for seven days. The seed I planted by returning the small grant grew into a much more substantial relationship.

If we are not self-employed, then we have a responsibility to our employer as well. We show integrity when we take the time to understand the local rules and regulations and then abide by them. If the local policy is to complete all test reporting by 6:00 p.m. daily, we show integrity by doing our best to have them all completed. Just because we are providers does not mean we get special dispensation from the local rules and customs. If you disagree with a policy, work through established channels to change it. There is nothing wrong with advocating for change, but being insubordinate demonstrates a lack of integrity and will rarely lead to any positive change. Think about those who work with you. Whom do you respect more: the nurse who has your chart ready and complete before every patient visit or the one who always forgets to update the med list and retrieve the lab results? We are subject to the same perceptions!

What If You Have Compromised Your Integrity?

We probably all know providers who have compromised their integrity. The most egregious cases are nationally highlighted in major lawsuits or press releases. Most, however, are a lapse in judgment during an otherwise unremarkable career. Maybe they are precipitated by financial stress or emotional distress, but the result is the same. In some cases, licenses or hospital privileges are lost while in others, they are not. Fortunately, this is one area where our healthcare systems appear to function well. There are well-established protocols to deal with disruptive providers or those who have substance abuse issues. State medical boards have established policies and protocols for license removal and reinstatement. Medical staff bylaws likewise have established policies. Once there has been financial malfeasance or substance abuse, the process is pretty clear. More importantly, providers must recognize the warning signs and seek help before crossing the line. We are not immune to the stresses of life; if anything, we get an extra helping! It is perfectly acceptable for us to get help ourselves. Seek out the provider assistance programs at your institution. Do this before you become compromised. There is no shame in admitting to the stresses we all feel! We deserve nothing less than the care we give our patients.

If you have been reading between the lines, you know that I have not always been a model citizen. I never crossed the integrity line, but I certainly needed help with relationships and dealing with work stress. I have been referred to the local hospital counselor, and I have independently sought out life coaching and professional coaching. These experiences have helped me grow and avoid a major meltdown.

While this book is not about burnout, I am certainly aware of the many providers suffering from this syndrome. I encourage you to seek a coach or counselor to help you. This is not a sign of weakness. Rather, you respect yourself and are willing to make changes as needed. In my mind, this is true integrity. While compromising financially or professionally is not good, compromising our personal health integrity is worse!

One of the truest tests of integrity is its blunt refusal to be compromised.
—Chinua Achebe[24]

Steps You Can Take

Recommit to the vows you took when you first became a provider.

Remind yourself daily that you must resist the temptation to do anything that is remotely unethical (even if it might be legal).

Be particularly aware of your actions and interactions when you are tired or frustrated.

Remember that your actions outside the hospital are just as important as those within the hospital.

If you are emotionally stressed, burning out, or in financial duress, please seek out professional help.
You can start at your primary institution. They have established resources to assist you. You can also find a life coach or counselor in the community. I will discuss this in more detail in chapter 13.

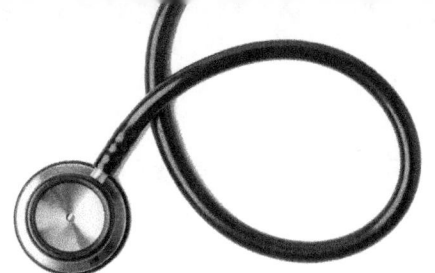

Chapter 12

Accountability

Accountability for Patient Safety

As providers, we have much to be thankful for. But to whom much is given, much is also required. One of those requirements is accountability. We are granted the right to make life-altering decisions for our patients. We are also human and fallible. Despite our best efforts and the most well-planned safeguards, mistakes will happen, and iatrogenic errors will occur. How we handle those events is a window to our character. Do we take account, or do we shift the blame? Do we self-reflect, or do we downplay and ignore?

I once was called to an emergency situation that highlights the gut-wrenching reality of this dilemma. An elective operation resulted in a complication requiring the placement of a kidney drainage tube after surgery. The patient was extubated after the original surgery and then transferred to the imaging suite for the nephrostomy tube placement. During the tube placement, the very obese patient was placed on her stomach and repeatedly sedated due to complaints of severe pain. It was late afternoon. One provider and four nurses were attending to the patient, having been asked to stay after hours to perform this task. Once the procedure was complete and the patient undraped, it became obvious that the patient was cyanotic and not breathing. That's when I was called in a panic.

As I reviewed the monitor recordings from the procedure, I saw a clearly documented, gradual, and dramatic decline in the patient's oxygen saturation followed by bradycardia. During the resuscitation efforts, myriad potential explanations were offered up including some undetected cardiac issue, a massive pulmonary embolus, or a medication reaction. The truth, unfortunately, was oversedation to the point the patient stopped breathing. No one had taken accountability for monitoring the patient and ensuring her safety during the procedure. Nor did anyone want to own up after the fact. It was a perfect storm: an add-on procedure, late afternoon, an obese patient, a new technician on the monitoring station, and an operator who was there infrequently (i.e., no team dynamic).

> Despite our best efforts and the most well-planned safeguards, mistakes will happen, and iatrogenic errors will occur. How we handle those events is a window to our character.

But as providers, the buck stops with us. It is our responsibility to be accountable to the patient and to ensure our team is likewise being accountable. Far better to immediately admit our honest oversight than to wait until the legal team is knocking on the door.

Accountability to Our Job, Colleagues, and Families

Not all accountability is life-altering. Accountability can be as simple as signing that verbal order you told the nurse you would sign. It can be showing up on time for the family conference you asked the ward clerk to arrange. Perhaps you will have to return home to collect the pager you left on the counter by mistake rather than hope no one needs you while you go to the movies. Accountability also means abiding by local policy and procedure even when you may disagree. You can work to change it later, but for now, you are accountable to it. I once had to discipline a physician who believed he was exempt from our infection policy forbidding wearing street clothes in the procedure room. He felt the rule was silly and that it was too time-consuming in his busy schedule for him to bother changing!

We must demonstrate accountability with our colleagues and families as well. When your partner is an hour late to relieve you from your shift, they are not being accountable. When you promise to cover for your partner during their son's birthday party but forget, you are not being accountable. When you promise to take a second look at a complicated case but put it off, you are not being accountable. I struggled with being accountable to my wife and children. For years Dinah asked me to call home at 5:00 p.m. so that she could have a sense for when I might get out of work and plan accordingly. For years I did not take that request seriously. I had many good reasons, but they were just excuses for me not being accountable to her request and my promise. And when I did finally start calling every day at 5:00, it took several more years for me to accurately estimate when I might actually leave for home! It took even longer for my wife to believe me.

Accountability for Our Training

As Stephen Covey says, "Accountability breeds response-ability."[25] When we are being accountable, we must respond to events in our lives. As providers confronted with problems, we are expected to have answers and to have them quickly! Most providers have witnessed a code blue situation where CPR is being performed and resuscitation of a patient is being attempted. I have witnessed well-run codes where the provider responded clearly and with authority. I have also witnessed codes where the provider was timid and indecisive. We all have to have advanced cardiac life support training. It becomes clear in these code situations who takes it seriously; in other words, who is accountable for the information being taught. Those who are accountable for the material taught, as Covey puts it, are able to respond appropriately under pressure.

We must also maintain our general knowledge and skills. Most states and institutions have CME requirements. Many also have focused practice performance evaluations (FPPE). It is easy for our knowledge to erode due to lack of use. Compound this with the new knowledge being added daily to our field. Few health systems provide ongoing opportunities for continuing education. Certainly, we can take time off to go to a conference, but for the most part, our continued learning depends on our initiative and is done during our off time. When I have worked in academic institutions, the trainees and the required lectures have served to keep me up to date. In nonacademic settings, I have had to develop other reference materials. Fortunately, with the internet, it is now easy-to-find information.

My former department of medicine chair, Dr. William N. Kelley, would quiz us if we had not researched anything we did not fully understand: "Did you eat yesterday? If so, then you had time to look that up!" Back then, we went to the library and read about it in a book. I'm not advocating such a strict policy, but his words are a constant reminder to me that we are accountable to keep up on issues in our field and to research patient problems that we do not fully understand. Be a lifelong learner. Doing so is easy in today's digital world and pays big dividends for your patient care.

Accountability in Culture

Accountability can be enhanced or degraded by the culture in which we practice. "If you are building a culture where honest expectations are communicated, and peer accountability is the norm, then the group will address poor performance and attitudes," says Henry Cloud.[26] I have certainly found this to be true. When I was in training, Dr. Kelley created that culture. The environment he supported set expectations and fostered accountability in the training program. We young physicians were taught the importance of being professional in how we dressed and how we interacted, researching things we did not understand, being punctual, comprehensive handoffs, and teamwork. The senior residents felt the weight of accountability for the interns and patients under their care. By the time we graduated, we had learned how to carry that weight. The culture demanded that we did.

I have also experienced a different training culture. At one time I practiced at a large community teaching hospital. The training program there was quite different from what I had experienced as a resident. Oversight was provided by physicians with community practices. Thus, they were only at the hospital sporadically. The program director was a perfunctory position. Resident supervision and evaluation were nearly nonexistent. In fact, most evaluations were fabricated just before the Accreditation Council for Graduate Medical Education (ACGME) inspections. Even the bare minimum lectures or rotations needed to satisfy the ACGME regulations were often not met. Most importantly, the residents never learned how to carry the weight of accountability and responsibility. Instead, they learned how to keep the attending physicians happy and get by with the least amount of energy. There was no culture of responsibility for learning or for competence.

After graduation, many of these residents ended up drifting from one position to another. Very few were competitive enough to secure fellowship positions. Many took hospitalist positions. Sadly, several of these people committed suicide during the first months of their independent practice under the stress of new positions that called on them to perform at a level they had never experienced and were unprepared to tackle. Hospitalists routinely admit and discharge five to ten patients daily while caring for a census of at least twenty patients. It is not easy! I once helped start a hospitalist program at a small institution. I had not been that exhausted since my internship year, but I was lucky—I had a strong foundation from my own training.

We providers must take responsibility to create a culture that expects and encourages excellence, celebrates training, and enables continued learning to be enjoyable, not just another mandated exercise. If we practice in a training facility, our most important role is to ensure that the trainees are accountable for learning how to practice independently. This seems obvious, but too often, trainees are not pushed to grow and develop independently. While limiting work hours or numbers of patients cared for may make the role less physically demanding, it does not build accountability. Do you think you can train for running a marathon race by running only one mile daily for training? Of course not! Why do we believe we can train providers who will have to care for twenty patients at once by limiting them to the care of only three?

If you practice in a nonteaching environment, you can encourage accountability with your colleagues to some degree, but the responsibility is best handled by the hospital system or medical staff office. On the other hand, you can easily encourage accountability with your office staff and with the hospital staff you interact with. Using the principles of teaming, equity, community, and honor, you can develop a culture of accountability with your staff. It may take time, but it will happen with clear expectations, appropriate training, honest feedback, and debriefing sessions. It will not happen by itself, however. This effort needs a champion. In my opinion, that champion should be the provider or a group of providers with like-minded goals.

Let me share a personal example of creating accountability with hospital staff. I was never formally trained to read echocardiograms. I was exposed to these studies repeatedly but always had colleagues who formally interpreted them. When I began working in smaller hospitals, I had to learn how to interpret these studies myself. Fortunately, I found some great, easy-to-understand books and fantastic websites for training and reference. However, the most important way that I learned was by working with the sonographers at the hospital. I called them nearly daily to ask about specific studies and specific calculations. Together, we researched the best ways to assess certain conditions. We worked to keep each other sharp and up to date on the latest advancements in the imaging equipment and the analysis tools. We created a culture that fostered further investigation, encouraged research, and expected function on the cutting edge. Individually, we could not have been as effective, but together, it was intellectually stimulating and fun! This also created a two-way accountability culture. They knew I was looking at their work and were concerned that we get the right information for the patient. I knew they were expecting me to spend time looking over their studies and that they reviewed my interpretations to see if we differed. It was a classic win-win-win situation. I improved, they improved, and the patient got accurate test results!

Providers are granted great responsibility. One of our most important responsibilities is to create a culture of accountability. This will be a lifelong, critically important endeavor. We are all quite busy, but I encourage you to look for opportunities to help others in the system be more accountable. Ultimately, this breeds greater efficiency, fewer errors, and better patient care. Seize these opportunities to be a leader. You are in a unique position to do so.

Steps You Can Take

Focus on your training.
By being accountable for what you need to learn, you will be better able to respond when called upon. Spend time learning something new daily.

If you make a mistake, own it.
Be accountable for your actions. Honest mistakes are forgivable; blame shifting and cover-ups are not!

Remember that you function as part of a team—model accountability for them by being punctual and professional.

If you work in a larger system, work to raise the cultural level of accountability.
This will take time, but if you don't take the lead, who will?

Ensure that your patient care handoffs are complete and accurate.

Look for opportunities to create a culture of accountability, especially with your office and hospital staff.

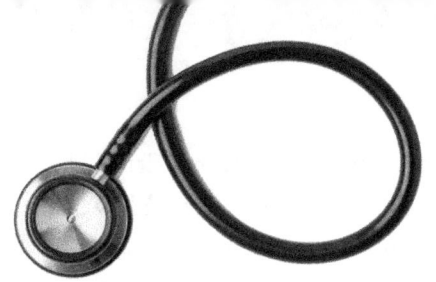

Chapter 13

Leadership in Medicine

Leadership concepts are not taught to providers. Instead, we are filled with knowledge and protocols and unleashed into a world in which we are viewed as leaders but are wholly unequipped to act like them. Despite the talk of some people being born leaders, there are very few effective leaders who did not receive training. Training could come in college classes but more often occurs in dedicated mentoring and experiential settings. For example, a friend of mine once worked for Ford Motor Company. He was brought into their leadership track. Approximately every two years, he was moved to a different department in the company—a few years in sales, a few years in marketing, a few years in accounting, and so on. He was even sent to South America to work in a branch of the company in Brazil. In each setting, he was mentored in the leadership skills needed to succeed and become well-rounded. It was on-the-job training, deliberate, and the company organized it. I have never heard of an intentional program such as this occurring during medical training. I believe we are worse off because of it.

Mentors

While a thorough review of leadership skills important to providers is beyond the scope of this book, I can highlight a few concepts that I have found helpful. Developing leadership skills is foreign to most providers. Nonetheless, we have all had influential persons acting as mentors in our lives. I remember several mentors who were critical in my development. I have already mentioned William Kelley. He was an old-school educator from the days before work-hour rules. I recall not having updated a patient's problem list, and he asked if I had slept the night before! Since I had, in fact, gotten a few hours of sleep, he responded that I had time to do so. Joking aside, he modeled that we had a responsibility to be complete and as sure of our treatment plans as possible. On another occasion, he escorted me out of the room where we were holding the morning report. I was wearing scrubs. I became acutely aware that we were expected to dress the part and to care for ourselves as professional physicians. Even if we had been up all night, he expected us to shower and wear fresh clothes to start the next day! While dress codes have become more casual over the past decades, being professional in our appearance has not become optional. Residents on my service are required to wear clothes (not scrubs) when on duty during the day unless they are performing a procedure. Certainly, I have had many complaints at the time, but without fail, once they have graduated, they recognize the importance of this simple concept.

If you want to be respected as a leader by your patients and colleagues, demonstrating self-respect for your appearance is a great start. Lest you think I am too old-fashioned, think of this for a minute: have you ever seen the president of the United States or a United States senator show up for a meeting in torn jeans and filthy sneakers? Have you ever seen a medical student interviewing for a residency job show up in torn scrubs, a filthy white coat, and a five-day beard? Of course not! Politicians are just debating how your tax money is spent; as a provider, you are about to impact someone's future functional ability or life! If you want your patients to respect you, you need to look respectable. Dr. Kelley not only taught me medicine, but he also taught me several leadership principles. We are accountable to be knowledge-able about our patients, and in holding a responsible position of high esteem, we need to act like it.

Recognize Leadership in Others

Another mentor, Marc Thames, was my first boss as a young physician. He taught me additional leadership principles. By his very hiring of me, he demonstrated that leaders recognize potential in their junior colleagues and encourage them to grow. I was fresh out of fellowship, but Marc made me the catheterization laboratory director at the largest VA hospital in the country. He encouraged my research interests, provided protected time for me, and assisted me in obtaining research grants. He encouraged my interactions with industry while at the same time schooling me in the ethics of research and conflicts of interest. And with his red pen in hand, he dedicated time to honing my writing skills. Granted, we had much more protected time back then, but leaders need to encourage the next generation even in today's busy environment. We should always be grooming our replacements.

> We have a responsibility not just to complete as many billing activities as possible but also to transmit our medical and leadership knowledge to the next generation.

We have a responsibility not just to complete as many billing activities as possible but also to transmit our medical and leadership knowledge to the next generation. A good principle to follow is one of "three generations." By this, I mean you need a mentor who invests in you (generation one), to be working to improve yourself (generation two), and to be mentoring someone younger than you (generation three). Many of us have appreciated mentors, but few have been intentional about mentoring someone younger than us. The system has become so busy that this will require extra effort to establish. Do it anyway! You will not regret it.

Expand the Scope of Those Who Can Influence You

I have also learned leadership skills from more casual colleagues outside of my institution. I joined the Society for Cardiac Angiography and Interventions (SCAI) in the mid-1980s. This was prompted by

Dr. Frank Hildner, who was the editor of the society journal then. He rejected one of the first papers I submitted for publication. I was devastated and called him to object. He explained that the journal used a double-blind review process and that my rejection was not personal. He graciously invited me to join the society and to get involved in the peer-review process. And no, he did not accept my manuscript! After joining SCAI, I started volunteering for committees, participating in educational events and on writing groups, and getting to know more senior members. To my great surprise, twenty years later, I was approached about becoming SCAI president. I had no concept that I would be qualified or even noticed!

This experience taught me more important leadership principles. Leaders typically start at the bottom, serving on mundane committees and spending time around more senior colleagues. Leaders demonstrate commitment and faithfulness. Leaders are not afraid to do the work that is needed to advance a cause. Leaders remain humble. Providers who demonstrate these things will gradually be recognized as leaders. Leadership is not a title—it is an earned recognition, requiring time and conscious effort. Wearing a white coat does not make you a leader; what you do when you take it off does.

Learn about Your Natural Style

Part of earning leadership recognition is relationship building. This has been my Achilles' heel. I am a very task-oriented person. My personality tests consistently peg me as a strong D on the DISC model (more about that in a minute). In my drive to get things done, I have been blind to the interpersonal relationships critical to success. Sure, I can do it all myself, but effective leaders inspire others with vision and encourage them to be active participants in the process of achieving the goal. This has been a very hard lesson for me, one I continue to struggle with.

In my journey to improve this leadership trait, several tools have been invaluable. First, we need to understand our natural personality type. Several methods are available, but I recommend the DISC model as one that works well for professionals and aspiring leaders. You can take the assessment online for a minimal fee.[27] Once you understand your personality type, many of your behaviors will become clearer, and importantly, ways to overcome them or compensate for them can be explored. You will also learn important tips for how to relate to others who have different personality types. Trust me, this will save you many awkward interactions. *Please stop reading now and look into taking the assessment!*

The Benefit of Life Coaching

I highly suggest seeking out a qualified life coach to assist you in the journey. A recent study from the Mayo Clinic randomized eighty-eight physicians to either receive six coaching sessions or no coaching. Quality of life was assessed on a ten-point scale. The providers receiving coaching improved their quality-of-life scores by 1.3 points compared to only 0.1 points in the control group. Other measured variables—including burnout, resiliency, and emotional exhaustion—also improved to a greater degree in the coached group. They concluded that "professional coaching may be an effective way to reduce emotional exhaustion and overall burnout as well as improve quality of life and resilience for some physicians."[28]

When I accepted two of my prior jobs, I asked for professional coaching as part of the compensation package. In both cases, however, this coaching was directed more at accomplishing the goals I had set for the institution than building my leadership capabilities. This was a mistake. It would have been far better for me to have a leadership coach or a life coach! I did not suffer from an inability to get things done (remember, I am a strong D) but from knowing how to lead others. The Mayo study mentioned above involved life coaching, not task coaching. I sincerely wish I had been offered the same structured coaching opportunity early in my career. I think I could have avoided a number of potholes along the way. I feel so strongly about the importance of coaching that several years ago I became a certified life coach and have been mentoring a few younger colleagues. Doing so keeps me grounded and fulfills part of my three-generation responsibility.

Formal Leadership Training

In addition to life coaching, Harvard Business Review claims, "It's becoming clear that leadership training should be formally integrated into medical and residency training curricula."[29] It would be ideal to learn leadership skills in our training programs. In recent years, experiential programs to teach patient interaction and interview skills have been incorporated at medical schools. While these experiential programs may teach listening skills or specific physical exam skills, they do not teach leadership. Most training programs struggle to include all necessary medical knowledge and have no margin to include what is considered a nonessential skill set. Personally, I believe establishing solid leadership skills and principles would be far more valuable. We can look up medical facts. Treatment regimens are constantly changing and evolving. The internet provides nearly endless capability to find information. Far better to teach young providers how to think critically, manage their stress, and interact with others in difficult situations.

I did participate in a six-month "leadership" training at an academic institution. As it turned out, the intent was for us to become better at interacting with patients and companies who may wish to donate to the institution's foundation. We worked in small groups and developed proposals to support worthy causes or needs at the institution. The group interactions were good, but it was not leadership training. I participated in a second course with the word *leadership* in the title. This course was focused on how to better communicate with patients and direct the visit so that the patient's satisfaction with the visit would be enhanced. Of course, patient satisfaction is important, and the intent was admirable, but the course was not about personal leadership. I mention these examples as a caution. Not every offering with the word *leadership* in the title is about personal leadership skills. You will have to be discerning in evaluating the offerings.

Until leadership training is incorporated into provider training or continuing professional development, we are left to seek out this training independently. I strongly suggest that all providers enroll in some form of leadership training. Several specific organizations can be of assistance. The American College of Physicians offers the ACP Leadership Academy.[30] The American Association for Physician Leadership offers certificate and master's level programs.[31] Becker's Healthcare has compiled a list of courses offered by leading healthcare institutions.[32] Make an investment in developing your leadership skills. You will struggle to find the time for online courses or occasional in-person events, but it will be worth it considering you will have a forty-year-plus career.

Leadership Self-Development

Even if you do not enroll in a formal course, everyone can apply leadership skills to their own development. As John Maxwell encourages, we will be moving forward as long as we focus on two things: First, learn a new skill every year. It does not matter what it is; just engage in learning something new. A year ago, I taught myself how to do Excel pivot tables and dashboards. This year I am learning pickleball! Second, commit to grow in a personal character issue. This could involve counseling, reading, or courses designed to help you improve yourself in an area of weakness.[33] For me, it has been learning to listen more intently. Engage a significant other or a friend to be a mirror for you. Be intentional and monitor your progress.

At the risk of repeating myself, I believe that to heal the healthcare system, there needs to be an investment in providers. Like any successful enterprise, a system that invests in developing provider leaders and encourages integrity, accountability, and community will deliver a better product. In our case, that translates into better patient care. Encouraging provider leadership can lead to a more stable workforce, fewer complications, better efficiency, and better public relations. While providers can work toward this independently, a far more enjoyable and effective way is a partnership with the healthcare system. At one large system I worked in, providers were empowered, supported, and encouraged to develop optimal treatment plans and to use optimal procedures, devices, and test methods. Certainly, some of the optimal strategies were more expensive, but the system saved money through fewer complications and higher efficiency over time. It is time for all healthcare systems to recognize the vital role of provider leadership rather than assuming all leadership resides in business-school trained administrators. We can work synergistically to be better than either functioning independently!

Steps You Can Take

Seek out mentors in your practice environment.
Don't be afraid to ask a more senior provider for insight. They will likely be honored and thrilled to help you!

Seek out a younger colleague that you can mentor.
This could be someone in high school considering a medical career, a junior colleague from your prior residency, or a new provider joining your current group. Ask them if they would be interested. I suspect you will get a heartfelt "yes!"

Take a personality assessment, such as the DISC.
DISC refers to four personality dimensions: Dominance, Influence, Steadiness, and Conscientiousness. As Dave Beuhring puts it in terms of animals: Lions, Otters, Golden Retrievers, and Beavers. As human examples, you can expect a company CEO to be a strong D type. A politician is typically a strong I type. A strong S type is the person in your office organizing the social and community activities, and the C type is your accountant. Medical providers could be any of the four types. The way you function in the healthcare environment will be vastly different. Again, I strongly encourage you to take the assessment online for a minimal fee.[34]

Hire a life coach experienced in professional development and leadership.
The Physician Coaching Institute is a good place to start looking.[35]

Enroll in a formal physician leadership course.
The American College of Physicians offers the ACP Leadership Academy.[36] The American Association for Physician Leadership offers certificate and master's level programs.[37] Becker's Healthcare has compiled a list of courses offered by leading healthcare institutions.[38]

Consciously work on a new skill and strive to grow personally.
No financial cost, but huge leadership benefits!

Encourage your healthcare system to invest in provider leadership programs.
Work through your medical staff office to build consensus.

Part Four

Implementing Changes

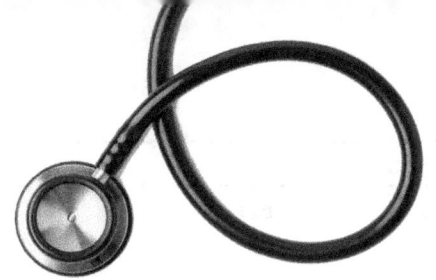

Chapter 14

What Would It Look Like to Be Fulfilled Again?

Let me take the liberty to paint a picture of a potential future state where providers are once again passionate about delivering healthcare, enjoy going to work every day, and feel that their efforts are appreciated. I'm going to do this in the form of a short story set in the fictional town of Pleasantville, a blue-collar working town somewhere in the Midwest. The local hospital, Pleasantville Charity Hospital (PCH), has one hundred licensed beds and an average census of about seventy-five patients. The hospital owns the multispecialty provider group and has an attached office building where over 80 percent of the providers practice. About eighty miles to the north is Megatown, a thriving city of close to one million persons. Megatown General Hospital (MGH) is recognized as the regional tertiary care center and operates with an employed provider base.

Most MGH providers also hold positions at the Founder's University School of Medicine. The cast of characters is set (I assure you I made all of these up), so let's see what a few typical days have in store for the providers at PCH and MGH.

Cast of Characters
Megatown General Hospital (MGH)
Dr. Mac Hart: Cardiologist
Dr. Tom Green: Fellow
Ms. Janice Ballard: Nurse Practitioner
Mr. Sammy Alemu: Physician's Assistant
Ms. Carole Billip: Charge Nurse in Coronary Care Unit
Dr. Phillip Jackowitz: Medicine Resident
Drs. Bonner and Levey: Senior Residents
Ms. Paula Espy: Housekeeper
Dr. Jamal Umpuno: Hospitalist
Dr. Id Mufassa: Emergency Department Physician
Ms. Lacretia Jones: Dr. Hart's Office Manager
Mr. Tommy Mancini: Dr. Hart's Office Nurse
Dr. William Barnes Jr.: Chief Medical Officer
Mr. Sanjay Patel: President
Pleasantville Charity Hospital (PCH)
Dr. Brenda Mostow: Internist
Mr. TJ Clark: Nurse Practitioner
Ms. Bethany Etsey: Charge Nurse on ward 3W
Dr. Stephanie Vespa: Hospitalist
Ms. Kayla Brownstone: Dr. Mostow's Office Nurse
Mr. Benjamin Unser: Dr. Mostow's Office Manager
Dr. Margo Zendi: Chief of Staff
Ms. Angela Bennito: President of PCH
Mrs. Melissa Clark: Billing Specialist and IT at PCH
Ms. Peg Zolden: Case Manager at PCH

Mrs. Mary Chaudhry arrived at about 5:00 a.m. at the emergency room at PCH, having agreed to go only after her daughter and son-in-law physically removed her from the recliner and carried her to the car. Unfortunately, she is a frequent visitor to PCH. She is also a regular visitor to MGH and had been discharged only ten days previously, having been cared for by Dr. Mac Hart, a cardiologist. PCH has a semiofficial relationship with the tertiary center in Megatown. They share the same electronic medical record, and MGH has agreed to provide specialty services for them in a timely fashion. They have established a directory of hotline or back-office phone numbers enabling rapid direct communication between providers at the two centers.

Dr. Brenda Mostow is Mrs. Chaudhry's primary care physician and works closely with the heart failure team at MGH to care for her advanced ischemic cardiomyopathy. Tommy Mancini is a nurse in Dr. Hart's office and runs the advanced heart failure service. He provides a minimum of weekly updates to Dr. Mostow, or more frequent updates if the patient is at MGH or changing medication regimens. Much of this coordination happens between Tommy and Kayla (Dr. Mostow's nurse) at a nursing level, but everything is documented, and issues can be easily escalated to Drs. Hart and Mostow as needed.

Today, Mrs. Chaudhry admits that she has not wanted to take her diuretic for the past two days. She did not want to be running to the restroom all day when she was out shopping with her visiting out-of-town college roommate. Last night she couldn't sleep, even when sitting upright in her recliner. Luckily, her daughter Ariel checked on her before going to work and brought her in to be treated. The emergency physician assumed she would just need a bit of diuresis and arranged for her to be admitted to Dr. Vespa, the hospitalist at PCH. Per their protocol, three things happened at 7:30 a.m.: Dr. Mostow was notified by secure message that her patient was admitted. Dr. Hart was notified that one of his heart failure oversight patients was admitted. Finally, both nurses, Tommy and Kayla, were messaged to close the loop. When Mrs. Chaudhry's daughter called Dr. Mostow's office for an update, Nurse Kayla was not surprised and could easily update her. A three-way call had been arranged by late morning by Charge Nurse (CN) Bethany Etsey. Drs. Hart, Vespa, and Mostow spoke for only three minutes, but all agreed on a plan for attempted diuresis for forty-eight hours with subsequent transfer if the patient did not improve.

Dr. Vespa cared for Mrs. Chaudhry for the next few days, but Dr. Mostow stopped over a few times to encourage her patient and stay up to date on the progress. Dr. Mostow was busy, to be sure, but her schedule had built-in wiggle room to accommodate such inpatient visits and the occasional add-on urgent visit in clinic. Dr. Mostow and Nurse Practitioner (NP) TJ at her office had become very efficient. Dr. Mostow has worked with NP TJ ever since he'd graduated from nurse practitioner school. For years, she had encouraged him to learn more and grow in his ability to take on independent responsibility. They met throughout the day to discuss difficult or interesting cases. He could easily cover for her if she needed to run to the hospital. And she could cover for him when he needed to be out or run an urgent personal errand.

Dr. Mostow was in office 201 on the corner of the professional building. Her name was on the door. She had dressed the space in an upbeat but professional decor. All her office staff were trained in basic customer service. How they treated the patients was an integral part of their performance evaluation. It was clear in the office that the patient's needs came first and that their job was to serve the patient no matter how trivial. Every morning started with a group meeting. The various staff (including Dr. Mostow and NP TJ) rotated turns bringing in a simple morning snack, perhaps specialty coffee, sometimes breakfast pizza, not too often doughnuts. During these times, they not only reviewed the upcoming patient schedule but also supported each other. Everyone knew that Nurse Kayla was trying to get pregnant. They knew that Office Manager Benjamin's fiancée was two hundred miles away finishing her master's program in social work. They knew that NP TJ's wife, Melissa, also worked at PCH in the billing office. This morning, Dr. Mostow told the team about her upcoming trip to Orlando with her grandchildren.

About once every two weeks, Dr. Margo Zendi (chief of staff at PCH) would drop in and enjoy a piece of breakfast pizza. She had been instrumental in establishing the collaboration between PCH and MGH. She had been elected chief of staff for the past fifteen years.

She knew all the providers and was a staunch advocate of delivering quality care at a local level. She had worked with United Medical Care Insurance to develop the outcomes-based payment schedule. United covered about 60 percent of the workers in Pleasantville. Since implementing this scheme, overall hospital admissions had fallen by 15 percent, and readmissions for congestive heart failure were down from 25 percent to 12 percent. All the primary providers at PCH participated in an evidence-based tracking system for major medical conditions. Success was measured by how well they met these evidence-based criteria, not how many office visits they could squeeze into an afternoon.

Melissa, who handled billing at PCH, had enjoyed the transition to outcomes-based payment. Instead of fighting United every day to get specific services covered, she could spend time creating dashboards and tracking systems that measured the health of their patients. Dr. Zendi had tapped her to lead that clinical informatics development. As a bonus, NP TJ could provide clinical context whenever needed! The providers at MGH also appreciated this payment system. For example, Dr. Hart traveled to PCH twice a month to oversee a local heart failure clinic. His expertise was directed toward particularly difficult or complicated patients. No one cared that he didn't have a rapid-fire patient visit schedule. His ability to interface with the local providers and provide continued training and specific tips and tricks resulted in a measurably lower hospitalization rate for heart failure patients in Pleasantville and an improved profit margin at PCH for the United Medical Insurance patients. On the days when Dr. Hart was in town, they typically held a lunch meeting where he provided up-to-date information on various cardiology topics for the hospitalists and primary care providers. Ms. Angela Bennito, president of PCH, always attended and was happy to provide a nice catered lunch.

Back in the hospital (PCH), CN Bethany gathered Dr. Vespa and the other team members for morning rounds. CN Bethany oversaw the thirty beds on ward 3W. She worked every weekday starting at 7:00 a.m. Her counterpart, CN Julie, worked on the weekends. They would meet virtually on a Zoom call on Friday and go over the patient situation. Between the two of them, ward 3W was always running smoothly. CN Bethany did the scheduling, and she worked hard to develop a fluid and responsive schedule. She preferred everyone to work ten-hour shifts, but she also had several nurses who had outside lives that were more flexible.

Today, Carl was the nurse taking care of Ms. Chaudhry. When it was time to round on her, Nurse Carl joined CN Bethany and the rest of the team. Dr. Vespa gave a quick medical update and outlined the plan she had developed with Drs. Hart and Mostow. Rounding with them were the 3W social worker, Areny, and the case manager, Peg. Once a week, PCH president Ms. Bennito would join them. She and Dr. Zendi felt it important to experience how frontline care was delivered in their facility. Not infrequently, Ms. Bennito would send other members of the leadership team for a day of rounding. At the monthly administrative staff meetings, a standing agenda item was to report their experience during hospital rounds. Those discussions were often lively and resulted in many innovative ideas. Being immersed in the day-to-day care kept the leadership grounded in the hospital's primary mission.

The average length of stay at PCH was just under three days. Since most nurses were working four ten-hour shifts, it was common that a single nurse could care for the same patient throughout their inpatient stay. The nurse-patient relationship governed staffing assignments. If one nurse had more patients, then support staff (aides, volunteers, students) schedules were flexed to help them. For occasional special circumstances, schedules were shifted to allow the same nurse to continue to care for the patient. Since this was a cultural norm on 3W, nurses went out of their way to make it happen. When continuity was not possible for every patient, the less ill and more-likely-to-be-home-soon patients were assigned the new nurse. The more complex patients got priority for continuity.

Of course, Dr. Vespa had days off as well. She worked seven-day shifts. Her colleague worked the opposite seven-day shift. A third partner occasionally covered when someone was on vacation. They had committed to maintaining as much continuity as possible. Thus, one-to two-day coverage situations were frowned upon and rarely occurred.

On the changeover day, a full two hours was scheduled for a warm handoff. They reviewed each patient and went over the treatment plan in detail during this time. They enjoyed discussing difficult cases and catching up on how prior patients had done after they went off service. Similar, although briefer, handoffs occurred each evening when the nocturnist came on duty. More important was the handoff the following morning. The nocturnist made rounds with Dr. Vespa on the newly admitted patients before going home. This ensured a warm handoff and alerted the day staff to patient acuity. It also avoided the delay in getting testing started that is so frequent with overnight admissions. Those decisions were made jointly between the nocturnist and Dr. Vespa at the start of the day.

Today, during rounds on Mrs. Chaudhry, it was clear that she needed more education and support at home. The case manager arranged for Nurse Kayla to stop at the end of the day, go over the importance of medication compliance, and offer suggestions on how to handle medications while being active outside the home. They determined that either Nurse Tommy or Nurse Kayla would call her every day for a few weeks to reinforce this. The heart failure team had established an easy-to-access database that allowed any team member to see which patients needed special attention. Peg, the case manager, also arranged some home health nurse visits to organize a pill reminder system. That evening Nurse Carl was able to update Mrs. Chaudhry's daughter about the plan.

On rounds the next day, Nurse Carl was disappointed to report that Mrs. Chaudhry had not lost any weight, her urine output had been falling, and her renal function was deteriorating—not what anyone had hoped for. Dr. Vespa texted Dr. Hart for advice.

Up at MGH, Dr. Hart was the attending in the Cardiac Intensive Care Unit. He would be there for fourteen days. Dr. Green (cardiology Fellow) and medical resident Dr. Jackowitz would also be with him for fourteen days. MGH had worked with Founder's University and the graduate medical office to create a unique residency call schedule that allowed for enough mandated time away from work but did not sacrifice the important training experience obtained through patient continuity. Medical resident Phil Jackowitz would work every day until 6:00 p.m. He would care for his patients every day. His patients would be those he admitted or those for whom he was the initial daytime resident. He would continue to care for them until discharge, even if they were no longer in the critical care unit. Dr. Hart would be their attending physician throughout their hospital stay and on call every night while on service to handle patient care questions. For emergency procedures, he shared call with two other staff physicians. This morning he was rounding on his sixteen ICU patients when the text came through. He texted Dr. Vespa back within a few minutes, advising her to hold the diuretics and start an infusion of dobutamine.

Rounds at MGH were not that different from the community hospital to the south. There was a defined team with Dr. Hart in charge. CN Carole rounded on every patient and coordinated having each patient's nurse available during rounds when they got to that patient. Physician Assistant (PA) Sammy Alemu was a critical care specialist who worked exclusively in the ICU and handled many of the lines and various support pumps and systems. NP Janice Ballard coordinated medical care and was an important liaison between the ICU, the emergency room, and the step-down unit. She particularly helped the patients as they transferred out of or into intensive care. Drs. Green and Jackowitz were there primarily to learn from Dr. Hart and were expected to gradually demonstrate more and more independent medical decision-making ability. Drs. Bonner and Levey were medical residents with Dr. Jackowitz, albeit one year senior to him. Between the three of them, they covered all the patients, and each was expected to contribute to the care of every patient, with primary responsibility for those they admitted.

This morning as they were rounding on their sixth patient, a seventy-eight-year-old man with recurrent ventricular tachycardia, they received a call from Dr. Id Mufassa in the emergency room. A helicopter was landing with a twenty-five-year-old woman in cardiogenic shock from suspected fulminant myocarditis. Dr. Hart dispatched Dr. Green and NP Ballard to the helicopter pad to meet the new arrival. He instructed Dr. Bonner to take over rounds and continue with CN Carole, PA Sammy, and the other two residents. Their first task was to open up a room for the new patient. Dr. Hart motioned to Paula from housekeeping, pretending to wash his hands in the air. She knew that was his signal that she would need to perform an emergency clean of the soon-to-be-vacated room.

Mr. Sanjay Patel, MGH's president, spent his morning rounding with the team. He was proud of the team and realized it was time for him to step back but be ready to help in any way needed. Dr. Hart made two more calls—one to Lacretia in the office to make his afternoon patients aware he could be delayed and one to the organ transplant coordinator. It was going to be a long day.

After the morning meeting in room 201, with freshly baked banana bread supplied by Nurse Kayla, Dr. Mostow's team was ready for their morning patient visits. Dr. Mostow and NP TJ worked a joint schedule, meaning they might each see every patient but for different parts of the visit. This was decided on the fly, dependent on patient needs. They kept four to five rooms busy, moving effortlessly from one to the next. Office Manager Benjamin and Nurse Kayla were always a few steps ahead, ensuring that needed lab results, outside records, accurate medication lists, and the like were ready when the providers arrived at the room. They typically allowed twenty to thirty minutes of prep time before every visit. The patients understood that this prep time was an important part of their visit. If their visit was scheduled for 10:30, they understood that they might not see the provider until 11:00. When patients needed lab work, it was drawn in the room. If in-office testing (for example, an electrocardiogram, spirometry, ankle-brachi-al-index, or a six-minute walk) was needed, it was done while they were there. All follow-up testing and visits were scheduled before the patient left the office. All patients left with an after-visit summary sheet, which both the providers and the staff reviewed with them.

Occasionally, Nurse Kayla got a call from a patient who was having an acute problem. Unless it was life threatening, they were always invited to come to the office. The fluid office system made it easy to work in an occasional urgent visit.

The providers had EHR stations readily available outside each room. They made a special effort not to use the computer while in the room with the patient, focusing rather on listening to what the patient was saying and then doing a thorough exam. They had optimized their EHR templates so that all but the most complex visits could be easily documented. The entire care team prided themselves on keeping the problem and history lists up to date and free of duplicates or errant entries. They had spent time standardizing their nomenclature. For example, patients with heart failure and a low ejection fraction had "heart failure with reduced ejection fraction (HFrEF)" listed on their problem list. They did not have entries such as "CHF," "heart failure," "systolic failure," or any other variation taking up real estate on the list. (As a resident, I remember when Chairman of Medicine William Kelley made rounds. He always looked for the problem list first. This list is a central component in communicating what is wrong with the patient and ensuring that nothing is overlooked. Remember, I learned this the hard way!)

The outcome dashboards developed by Melissa in billing were displayed in the exam room during each visit so that the providers could be reminded of the key metrics needing attention. Key educational literature was also readily available in each exam room, allowing the provider to personally give it to the patient and stress the importance of reading it. Occasionally, Dr. Mostow wanted some extra teaching by one of the staff. The patient could stay in their room, and the staff went to them for the additional reinforcement. By noon, the team had seen twenty patients, and all charting was complete.

Dr. Mostow opted to run to the hospital to see Mrs. Chaudhry before heading to the physician's lounge to meet Dr. Vespa for lunch. NP TJ was going to meet his wife, Melissa, for lunch in the food court. He was thinking that a trip to Orlando might be fun for them too!

Mrs. Chaudhry smiled when she saw Dr. Mostow enter the room. Dr. Mostow always grabbed a chair and sat when she visited patients. She wanted to convey to them that she was in no hurry and that they were important, which in her case was the truth! Mrs. Chaudhry had been her patient for ten years, ever since she first presented with a large myocardial infarction. Mrs. Chaudhry trusted her. Ariel, her daughter, trusted her. Dr. Mostow had always been straight with them, and they were well aware of the severity of Mrs. Chaudhry's situation. Mrs. Chaudhry looked at Dr. Mostow with a hint of moisture in her eyes and said, "I think I might not make it this time." Mrs. Chaudhry was scared.

Dr. Mostow took her hand and squeezed it. She nodded and said, "Maybe, but we have been here before, and you are a fighter! I know you don't want to, but we may have to transfer you to Dr. Hart up north to work his magic." Dr. Mostow asked about Ariel and her dog and the three grandkids. She even got a smile from Mrs. Chaudhry when they reminisced about the recent summer festival. Dr. Mostow gave her hand a final squeeze and rose, telling Mrs. Chaudhry that they would make a final decision on transfer later that afternoon once they could determine if the dobutamine was helping.

NP Janice called Dr. Hart a few minutes after the helicopter landed. Their new patient was indeed in cardiogenic shock and not looking too good. Dr. Hart activated the shock team. With CMO Dr. Barnes's full support, MGH providers had developed this specialized team so that complex multidisciplinary decisions could be made very rapidly with expert input. Team members included the ICU attending, a cardiothoracic surgeon, a cardiac anesthesiologist, a perfusionist, the transplant coordinator, and the lead case manager. Within five minutes, they assembled to assess the newly arrived patient and determine an initial action plan. She would need to be placed on a support system called ECMO, which included the ability to function for her lungs and her heart. Simultaneously, she would be registered in the national transplant database, just in case her heart did not recover using the support systems.

While Dr. Hart arranged the necessary procedures for the new patient, Dr. Bonner was progressing on rounds. Along with PA Sammy, CN Carole, and his fellow residents, the team had not missed a beat. This was Dr. Bonner's third year as a medical resident and his fourth month in the ICU. Dr. Hart and the other staff physicians had been working to prepare him for such a time as this. He had been expected to lead rounds under the oversight of Dr. Hart on many occasions. Today, he felt confident. His fellow residents knew their patients, and CN Carole and the other staff nurses respected his judgment. When things settled down, he would update Dr. Hart on each patient. During that update, Dr. Hart had the opportunity to teach further and encourage. Dr. Hart treated Dr. Bonner as a junior colleague and took a personal interest in ensuring he would be successful when he started his career. Previous residents called Dr. Hart now and then after they graduated, sometimes for advice, sometimes to thank him for the training and life-experience tips he had imparted to them.

PA Sammy worked with the surgeons and the perfusionists to get all of the ECMO equipment ready for the new patient. CN Carole arranged for the needed additional nursing staff required to care for a patient on ECMO and ensured that the case manager and social workers were aware that they would need to arrange emergency insurance coverage for the anticipated procedures. Everything was assembled in less than thirty minutes, and Dr. Hart went to work inserting the necessary tubes to initiate cardiopulmonary support. Once the patient was stabilized, he sought out the family and spent as much time as they needed to help them understand what was happening with their daughter. PA Sammy would stay near the new patient and provide updates to Dr. Hart as needed. The shock team would regroup later in the day to reassess the plan. But for now, Dr. Hart and his team had managed to get through rounds, manage a critically ill new patient, and coordinate care with their partner hospital to the south. Despite the unpredictable nature of the morning, they had not lost continuity, and their common goal had been maintained!

After lunch with Dr. Mostow, Dr. Vespa started her afternoon rounds. Nurse Carl had been updating CN Bethany on Mrs. Chaudhry's progress since starting the dobutamine. When Dr. Vespa stopped at the nursing station, CN Bethany gave her a quick update on all the patients. Together they determined how to attack the items needing attention. Some could be handled by the nurses alone, some needed social work or case management intervention, and some needed to be rechecked by Dr. Vespa personally. Frequent check-ins like this made it possible for Dr. Vespa to manage up to twenty patients at a time while still admitting new patients and discharging those ready to go home. By teaming together, they were able to avoid unnecessary prolonged stays, unanticipated financial issues, and many simple mistakes. This efficient flow prevented backups in the emergency department and saved the hospital significant money, especially for the patients covered by United Medical Care Insurance. Around 6:00 p.m., the nocturnal physician relieving Dr. Vespa arrived, and they spent forty-five minutes reviewing the current patients. The nocturnist was not just there to respond to emergencies and admit new patients—they were actively involved in ensuring the care plan for each patient was being executed. This was a key component to reducing the length of stay at PCH and was another way unnecessary mistakes were avoided. And importantly, Dr. Vespa could relax when she was off for the evening, knowing the patients were actively attended to.

The following morning, Dr. Vespa was rounding with the nocturnist on the new patients, Dr. Hart assembled his team for ICU rounds, and Dr. Mostow brought fresh fruit for her morning office meeting. Schedules were reviewed, patients were seen, families were reassured, and team meetings were held. Unfortunately for Mary Chaudhry, her kidney function continued to decline. Nurse Carl let CN Bethany and Dr. Vespa know that despite the dobutamine treatment, Mrs. Chaudhry's heart failure was not responding as hoped. As she had done a few days earlier, CN Bethany arranged a call between Drs. Hart, Mostow, and Vespa. On that call, they determined that

Mrs. Chaudhry would need to be transferred up to MGH for hemodynamic monitoring to guide further therapy.

Transfer between the two partner hospitals was far from the stressful task it had been ten years earlier. Nurse Tommy, in Dr. Hart's office, coordinated the necessary arrangements. Since their partnership agreement, the two facilities functioned more like one entity than two. They shared the same EMR, so it was more like transferring from one floor to another rather than to a different city. All the notes and medication information would be seamlessly reassigned to MGH. With one call, Nurse Tommy arranged for the ambulance to pick up Mrs. Chaudhry and bring her directly to the ICU at MGH.

Since Mrs. Chaudhry was covered by United Medical Care Insurance, her daughter was guaranteed two nights of lodging at the MGH hotel. Since many MGH patients were not local residents, Mr. Patel had pushed to build the attached hotel facility when he took over as president at MGH. The patients' families were distraught enough when a loved one was ill that searching for a place to sleep was the last thing they needed to worry about when they arrived in town. Since it was attached, the hotel also served as a long-term hospital "ward" for out-of-town patients who needed frequent medical procedures. These stable patients could stay at the hotel and come over as needed to the hospital for treatment. This worked wonders for transplant patients, radiation therapy patients, and the like. Insurers liked this arrangement as well. Paying for a hotel room was far less expensive than a standard hospital room!

Mrs. Chaudhry arrived at MGH around noon. Dr. Green met her when she arrived, ensured that the needed EMR information was available, and then assigned her care to Dr. Jackowitz. Once Dr. Jackowitz had seen her, he talked to Dr. Green, and they agreed to proceed with the hemodynamic monitoring. PA Sammy assisted the doctors in placing the needed monitoring catheters and getting Mrs. Chaudhry settled. After the initial measurements were performed, Dr. Hart met with Drs. Green and Jackowitz to go over the results and determine the next steps. It would be Dr. Jackowitz's job to execute these next steps. Dr. Green would be there for backup if needed.

Meanwhile, CN Carole had assigned Mrs. Chaudhry's nurse. This nurse would be with Mrs. Chaudhry for the next four days at a minimum. She and Dr. Jackowitz were Mrs. Chaudhry's primary team and responsible for keeping CN Carole and Dr. Hart updated whenever necessary. Later that afternoon, Dr. Mostow called Mrs. Chaudhry's room to check in and let her know she would be keeping up to date from Pleasantville.

Dr. Hart had devoted much of the morning to the young woman with cardiogenic shock. The shock team had met the night before and again this morning. The patient was listed in the national transplant database as potentially needing a heart transplant. The social worker and case manager had been successful in getting emergency insurance coverage for the unexpected expenses to come. The family had arrived and gotten a few hours of sleep at the MGH hotel. By afternoon, after twenty-four hours on the ECMO support system, things were starting to look a bit more hopeful. Everyone hoped that the young woman would recover on her own, but the system they had put in place was working. If she needed a transplant, all the necessary pieces were queued up and ready to go.

CMO Dr. Barnes even stopped by to see if he could help in any way. He was proud of the fifteen specialized response teams his support had enabled at MGH. In his mind, evidence-based, standardized responses that eliminated unnecessary variation were a key part of the excellent patient outcomes enjoyed by MGH. Others thought so as well. At least once a month, Dr. Barnes was invited to talk to other systems about the response team concept and how it had empowered his providers and given them a sense of ownership in the patient care process.

So . . . what happened during these theoretical few days at PCH and MGH? There was seamless care for a patient by her own primary care physician, an inpatient hospitalist, and a tertiary specialist. No one felt left out, and the focus was on the patient. Drs. Hart's and Mostow's office staffs were empowered to facilitate efficient care while building a sense of community at work. The residents at MGH were taught not just medical facts but also responsibility and independence. They were expected to succeed, and they rose to the occasion. Specialized teams effectively cared for critically ill patients in an orderly way. EMR systems worked to facilitate care, not impede it. Hospital administrators worked to support clinical providers and understand the issues in the trenches.

If this scenario sounds foreign, you are not alone. The simple changes and adjustments I have suggested in this book are not expensive, do not require outside consultants to initiate, and can be effective in nearly any environment. Whether you are a provider, an administrator, or anyone interested in improving our healthcare system, I suggest you are all capable of initiating change. All of us interact with others in the healthcare system. I would encourage you to take even one or two points I have outlined and try them in your own workplace. I think you will be pleasantly surprised at how even small efforts can make your workday more enjoyable. We all *need* to be rejuvenated. We all *can* be rejuvenated. For the sake of our patients, we all *must* be rejuvenated!

Take-Home Points

Drs. Hart and Mostow were the captains of their teams.
Their team members were consistent (if even for only two weeks at the teaching hospital). The team members all had a common goal.

Physician and nursing schedules were designed to provide continuity of care for the patients.
Whenever possible, the same nurse and the same physician cared for an individual patient throughout their hospital stay.

Provider schedules prioritized time for team meetings, unexpected patient needs, administrative tasks, and education.
For example, Dr. Hart was not expected to staff the outpatient clinic or the invasive laboratory while assigned to the ICU. Dr. Mostow's morning staff meeting was never cancelled.

Provider communication was emphasized.
Easy access between providers was enabled and an expected part of the day's activities.

Referring physicians, primary care physicians, and specialists collaborated on the care of their patients.
Notice that this took literally only minutes to accomplish, but it fostered a culture of collaboration.

Hospital administrators sought ways to encourage and support provider input in patient care pathways, quality improvement initiatives, and patient satisfaction.
There is no substitute for administrative participation in the daily delivery of care on the front lines. Such an experience naturally leads to collaboration.

Hospital administrators worked to create synergistic partnerships with other entities in the healthcare system.
They worked with provider groups, other facilities, and insurance companies to create systems that would enable patient care to be more efficient and provide better outcomes. These large-scale complicated agreements were the best use of their management training.

A sense of community was fostered between hospital administrators, providers, and support staff.
Notice that they worked alongside each other. They experienced care together. They honored each other's strengths.

Patients and their families were honored during the stressful healthcare challenges they faced.
A gesture of lodging, or a few focused minutes of eye-to-eye explanation goes a long way!

Provider activities were focused on improving patient care and ensuring continuity through the intelligent use of EMR systems and warm handoff protocols.
Continuity was king! Billing activity was a distant secondary goal.

About the Author

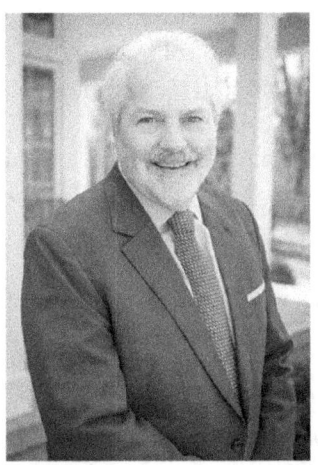

Dr. John McB. Hodgson is an internationally recognized cardiologist who has committed his career to improving the way healthcare systems work. He has experienced academic and community hospitals, multicity systems, small rural hospitals, private practice, and academic-employed practice. As a tenured professor of medicine, entrepreneur, inventor, and certified life coach, he has experienced varied approaches to healthcare in North America and around the world. He and his wife, Dinah, reside in Moreland Hills, Ohio.

In *Healing the System*, Dr. Hodgson draws on his experience to suggest simple, easy-to-implement changes that healthcare providers and administrators can make to combat the increasingly dysfunctional environment typical of current practice. These simple changes can bring a sense of fulfillment, joy, and satisfaction back to the practice of medicine. Not only will the providers of healthcare benefit, patients will also benefit, and the entire system will be energized.

Notes

1. "History And Development of CPT (Current Procedural Terminology)," CodingAhead.com, accessed March 21, 2022, https://www.codingahead.com/history-and-development-of-cpt-html/.

2. A. Baadh, et al., "The Relative Value Unit: History, Current Use, and Controversies." *Current Problems in Diagnostic Radiology* 45, (2016):128–132.

3. W. C. Hsiao, et al. "Resource-based Relative Values: An Overview." *Journal of the American Medical Association* 260, (1988): 2347–53.

4. Matthew R. Coffron and Carrie Zlatos, "Medicare Physician Payment on the Decline: It's Not Your Imagination." *Bulletin of the American College of Surgeons*, September 1, 2019. https://bulletin.facs.org/2019/09/medicare-physician-payment-on-the-decline-its-not-your-imagination/#printpreview.

5. "Catholic Church and Health Care," Wikipedia, accessed March 22, 2022, https://en.wikipedia.org/wiki/Catholic_Church_and_health_care.

6. Leslie Kane, "Death by 1,000 Cuts." Medscape National Physician Burnout & Suicide Report 2021, January 22, 2021, https://www.medscape.com/slideshow/2021-lifestyle-burnout-6013456#27.

7. "Handoffs Communication," Joint Commission Center for Transforming Healthcare, Improvement Topics, Accessed March 22, 2022, http://www.centerfortransforminghealthcare.org/projects/detail.aspx?Project=1.

8. Joe Cantlupe, "Expert Forum: The Rise (and Rise) of the Healthcare Administrator," AthenaHealth, November 7, 2017, https://

www.athenahealth.com/knowledge-hub/practice-management/expert-forum-rise-and-rise-healthcare-administrator.

9. E. J. Keller, et al., "The Growing Pains of Physician-Administration Relationships in an Academic Medical Center and the Effects on Physician Engagement," PLoS ONE 14, no. 2 (2019): e0212014. https://doi.org/10.1371/journal.pone.0212014.

10. Erin Mercer, "When Physician Leaders Work in Hospital Administration," Doximity Op-Med, July 30, 2019. https://opmed.doximity.com/articles/when-physician-leaders-work-in-hospital-administration?_csrf_attempted=yes.

11. Paul DeChant, "Building Bridges between Practicing Physicians and Administrators," An AMA StepsForward Module, May 20, 2021, https://edhub.ama-assn.org/steps-forward/module/2780305.

12. D. W. McMillan and D. M. Chavis, "Sense of Community: A Definition and Theory," *Journal of Community Psychology* 14, (1986):6–23.

13. What is the Sense of Community Index?" Sense of Community. https://www.senseofcommunity.com/soc-index/, accessed March 22, 2022.

14. Staff, "5 Common Physician Relations Faux Pas," *Becker's Hospital Review*, March 28, 2013, https://www.beckershospitalreview.com/hospital-physician-relationships/5-common-physician-relations-faux-pas.html.

15. Kenneth Bertka, "Leading Physician Engagement: Spanning Boundaries, Communicating Change," *Becker's Hospital Review*, March 25, 2013, https://www.beckershospitalreview.com/hospital-physician-relationships/leading-physician-engagement-spanning-boundaries-communicating-change.html.

16. Rose O. Sherman, "Building a Sense of Community on Nursing Units," *American Nurse*, March 11, 2013, https://www.myamericannurse.com/building-a-sense-of-community-on-nursing-units/

17. "Gallup's Employee Engagement Survey: Ask the Right Questions With the Q12 Survey," Gallup, accessed March 22, 2022, https://www.gallup.com/access/239210/gallup-q12-employee-engagement-survey.aspx.

18. M. Linzer, et.al. "Characteristics of Health Care Organizations Associated with Clinician Trust," *JAMA Network Open* 2, no. 6 (2019):e196201.

19. M. Linzer, et al. "10 Bold Steps to Prevent Burnout in General Internal Medicine," *J Gen Intern Med* 29 (2013):18–20.

20. "What is The Sense of Community Index?" accessed March 22, 2022, https://www.senseofcommunity.com/soc-index/.

21. M. Linzer, et al., "Working Conditions in Primary Care: Physician Reactions and Care Quality," *Annals of Internal Medicine* 151, (2009):28–36, W6–W9.

22. "Gallup's Employee Engagement Survey: Ask the Right Questions With the Q12 Survey," Gallup, accessed March 22, 2022, https://www.gallup.com/access/239210/gallup-q12-employee-engagement-survey.aspx.

23. Rick Warren, *The Purpose Driven Life: What on Earth Am I Here For?* Goodreads, accessed March 22, 2022, https://www.goodreads.com/work/quotes/2265235-the-purpose-driven-life-what-on-earth-am-i-here-for.

24. Chinua Achebe, BrainyQuote, accessed March 22, 2022, https://www.brainyquote.com/authors/chinua-achebe-quotes.

25. Stephen Covey, BrainyQuote, accessed March 22, 2022, https://www.brainyquote.com/authors/stephen-covey-quotes.

26. Henry Cloud, BrainyQuote, accessed March 22, 2022, https://www.brainyquote.com/authors/henry-cloud-quotes.

27. Professional Leadership–Online Profile, uniquelyyou, accessed March 22, 2022, https://uniquelyyou.org/catalog/online-profiles/disc-profiles/professional.

28. L. N. Dyrbye, et al. "Effect of a Professional Coaching Intervention on the Well-being and Distress of Physicians," *JAMA Internal Medicine* 179, (2019):1406–14.

29. Lisa S. Rotenstein, Raffaella Sadun, and Anupam B. Jena, "Why Doctors Need Leadership Training," *Harvard Business Review*, October 17, 2018, https://hbr.org/2018/10/why-doctors-need-leadership-training.

30. "ACP Leadership Academy," American College of Physicians, accessed March 22, 2022, https://www.acponline.org/meetings-courses/acp-courses-recordings/acp-leadership-academy.

31. "Leadership Programs," American Association for Physician Leadership, accessed March 22, 2022, https://www.physicianleaders.org/education/physicians.

32. Allison Sobzcok, "10 Key Leadership Programs for Physicians," Becker's ASC Review, December 30, 2015, https://www.beckersasc.com/asc-news/10-key-leadership-programs-for-physicians.html?oly_enc_id=7809H3426978E1B.

33. "Become the Leader You Were Born to Be," Maxwell Leadership, accessed March 22, 2022, https://www.johnmaxwell.com/.

34. Professional Leadership–Online Profile, UniquelyYou, accessed March 22, 2022, https://uniquelyyou.org/catalog/online-profiles/disc-profiles/professional.

35. "Become a Certified Physician Development Coach™," Physician Coaching Institute, accessed March 22, 2022, https://physiciancoachinginstitute.com/.

36. "ACP Leadership Academy," American College of Physicians, accessed March 22, 2022, https://www.acponline.org/meetings-courses/acp-courses-recordings/acp-leadership-academy.

37. "Leadership Programs," American Association for Physician Leadership, accessed March 22, 2022, https://www.physicianleaders.org/education/physicians.

38. Allison Sobzcok, "10 Key Leadership Programs for Physicians," Becker's ASC Review, December 30, 2015, https://www.beckersasc.com/asc-news/10-key-leadership-programs-for-physicians.html?oly_enc_id=7809H3426978E1B.

ORDER INFORMATION

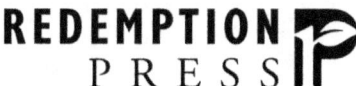
REDEMPTION PRESS

To order additional copies of this book, please visit
www.redemption-press.com.
Also available at Amazon, Christian bookstores,
and Barnes and Noble.

www.ingramcontent.com/pod-product-compliance
Lightning Source LLC
Chambersburg PA
CBHW071522180526
45171CB00002B/352